YES, you can!

Living and loving life with Type 1 diabetes

By Kristina Loskarjova

Copyright page
Yes, you can!

Copyright © By Kristina Loskarjova
ISBN: 978-1-8383828-9-6

All rights reserved.

No part of this book may be reproduced by any means, nor transmitted, nor translated into a machine language, without the written permission of the publishers.

Condition of Sale
This book is sold subject to the condition that it shall not, by way of trade or otherwise, be lent, re-sold, hired out or otherwise circulated in any form of binding or cover other than that in which it is published and without a similar condition including this condition being imposed on the subsequent purchaser.

Disclaimer
Every effort has been made to ensure that the information in this book is accurate and current at the time of publication. The author and the publisher cannot accept responsibility for any misuse or misunderstanding of any information contained herein, or any loss, damage or injury, be it health, financial or otherwise, suffered by any individual or group acting upon or relying on information contained herein. None of the opinions or suggestions in this book is intended to replace medical opinion. If you have concerns about your health, please seek professional advice.

Dedicated to Mum and Dad,
for their love, support and attention
from my earliest years.

FOREWORD

It is a great pleasure for a doctor to be able to recommend her patient's book, especially when she can read such an entertaining, thought-provoking perspective.

Is it hard to live with diabetes, or is it not? Is diabetes a disease or a lifestyle?

Kristina's book, which is filled with the inspiring life experiences of people with Type 1 diabetes, raises these questions, giving ideas on how to forge an advantage from the condition while describing all the 'hows' and 'whys'.

It was an exciting read for me, even though I've known and followed Kristina for 20 years.

My first memory of her is as a little girl with golden, curly hair and a startled look, who was supervised by an anxious mother. Yet throughout the years, we've learned a lot from each other during our coexistence: I taught her to understand diabetes, and she taught me its applicability in life.

I think it is very important to hear these stories from the patient's point of view, to understand how we can and should motivate ourselves and make diabetes our own.

Congratulations to Kristina! I recommend this book to all people living with diabetes and the providers who care for their health. It shows that it is not diabetes that leads our lives, but our lives that control diabetes. That's the real motivation!

Dr Almássy Zsuzsanna,
head doctor of the Metabolic Department
at Pál Heim National Institute of
Paediatrics in Budapest, Hungary

NOTICE

This book is intended strictly for motivational purposes and should not be perceived as medical advice. Everyone is different; we all have different bodies, different reactions and very different habits. If you wish to make changes to your treatment after reading any part of this book, you must consult and confirm the changes with your healthcare team first. The messages in this book are solely intended to help you in finding the joy and discipline in a new lifestyle and to show that, by following some simple habits, individuals with Type 1 diabetes can still do everything they ever wished to.

CONTENTS

Foreword v

Notice vii

Introduction 1

1 Your diagnosis: first steps 5

2 Telling others 21

3 Confidence 41

4 Eating out and in 55

5 Activities 71

6 Travelling 97

7 Careers 109

8 Nights out with friends 121

9 Mind, body and soul 137

10 Advice for parents of children with Type 1 diabetes 151

Afterword 161

Acknowledgements 163

Contributor biographies 165

Useful sources of further information: Local Diabetes Organisations And Charities 176

Author biography 177

INTRODUCTION

'I wish I could eat it… I wish I could do it… I wish I could be part of it…

If only I didn't have diabetes.'

This cry from the heart probably sums up the biggest fear people have when they are diagnosed with Type 1 diabetes. It's the fear of not being able to live a fulfilling life.

But let me reassure you right from the beginning: this fear is false!

I've spent 20 years with Type 1 and, having spent many of my formative years in the densely populated, fast-changing city of London, I've met countless individuals with Type 1. I've worked out that they fall into two categories. The first is people who tell me that they don't do certain things because they have diabetes. The best they can do is to treat it as a foe and fight it every single day. They have made a conscious decision to limit their lives and the things that they do. As a result, they feel beaten by diabetes. The second group is the polar opposite. These are people who do extraordinary things, day after day, *exactly because* they have diabetes. They break all the stereotypes and achieve everything others thought they couldn't. These heroes haven't just accepted their diagnosis and learned to treat diabetes as their friend – they've used it as the catalyst to boost the strong and happy personality they already have.

My aim in writing this book is to prove that *anyone* can live a wonderful life with diabetes today. Sure, if we found ourselves with this condition 100 years ago, things would've been very different, but nowadays there are a range of options that allow us to not only survive, but to prosper and live at least as well as everyone else. With this book I hope you will see that it is possible to cooperate with diabetes and live a very fulfilled life indeed.

Type 1s can do everything – from eating anything to undertaking challenging adventures to pursuing the most active sports.

Since I've been living with Type 1 from the age of 3, I think it is helpful to tell a lot of my own stories in this book. I've included them to give you some idea of what to expect growing up with Type 1, entering adulthood and beyond. I do understand that we are all individuals and everyone's story will be different. I just want to show that there is always a way around whatever challenges you might face – and, even when that way doesn't immediately always seem straightforward, a bit of humour goes a long way. I also understand that, as individuals, we all have different thoughts, concerns and priorities. It is for this reason that I recommend that you read this book in any way you like. Just because a book has a linear format, beginning at chapter one and working its way through to the end, it doesn't mean you have to read it that way. If you are planning a big trip and want to know about travelling with Type 1, go right ahead to chapter six. Likewise, if you're keen on sports, leap ahead to chapter five and read all about activities. The choice is entirely yours.

Rest assured, I am not painting an overly optimistic picture about Type 1. I have been realistic and not shied away from walking you through some of the hardships we might face when, say, eating out, meeting new friends or trying a new activity. The point is, though, it is all manageable. Yes, living with Type 1 can be, well, different, particularly when you compare yourself to people who don't have it. It can be hard sometimes too, when it destroys your daily plans and demands all your focus. And it can be scary, when your blood glucose is close to 0 and you realise you forgot your bag with your emergency food. But different is not all 'bad'. Different can be funny when your friends know the condition as well as you do and your daily blood checks become a bit like a comedy show. It can also be satisfying, when you eat your mum's sugary apple pie and stay within range.

Overall, Type 1 is not a big deal. If we remember the great things it has taught us, it feels like a superpower. The cost of this superpower is daily monitoring, constant concentration and inhuman responsibility. No holidays, no days off.

But hey, isn't that just what the life of a superhero is like?

You don't need to take my word for it. I have interviewed 17 Type 1 superheroes for this book. They come from all over the world and each one has a fantastic and inspiring story to tell. Whether it is achieving fame as an international music star, climbing mountains, racing cars or inspiring countless individuals as an influencer, they've done it all. What comes across in every case is that these people are all very different, very driven and genuinely happy.

Introduction

Right now, one out of every 430–530 people has Type 1 and the rates are showing a sharp uptick throughout the world. I am certainly meeting more and more people with the condition. I find that many people with Type 1, whether they are newly diagnosed or have had the condition for a long time, treat their condition as a disability. This should not be happening. Diabetes is not a disability – it is a perfectly manageable lifestyle.

Whether you are reading this book as someone who has just been diagnosed, as an experienced Type 1, as a parent, as a caring friend or just as a curious acquaintance, I hope that it helps you to understand a little bit more and that it widens your views on the potential of Type 1s. My hope is that, for Type 1s in particular, this book will be a source of motivation and help towards finding that all-important self-belief and inner power that will push you to explore the world. Diabetes should always be by your side as a friend and trustworthy companion, not as a mean enemy. And, if ever you feel a little lost, maybe this book will help you get on track again. Your life does not need to be restricted. The only borders you have are the ones your imagination sets up for you. At the very least, I hope that this book can shift your ideas about diabetes into a new perspective.

I will add one small caveat here. I am not medically trained, so no advice in this book should be perceived as medical. If you are looking for insights into the whys and wherefores of what is going on at the biological level, or the clinical options available to you to manage diabetes and keep your sugar levels stable, this is not the book for you. If this is what you are looking for, speak to your medical team and ask for their advice on information sources. A Google search will also lead you to a large number of very helpful websites that have a lot of the information you need. What I am offering here is a guide on how to live life with Type 1, gratefully, fearlessly and wholeheartedly. I am not an expert in diabetes management. I am an expert in life management for Type 1s!

Being a diabetic is a cool lifestyle that people should be proud of. There is no need to ever feel shy, awkward or ashamed of your condition. Am I a diabetic? *Yes.* I am and I am proud of it.

Whatever your reason for reading this book, I hope that by the end we will agree: life is equally exciting for everyone, including anyone with Type 1. In fact, it can be even more exciting because it can drive you on to do things other people only dream about.

1

YOUR DIAGNOSIS: FIRST STEPS

Yes, you can!

I vividly remember sitting in the doctor's office as he said, 'You have Type 1 diabetes. That means daily insulin shots for life. No more sugar from this point on at all.' I had a healthy lifestyle then, but his words were rough. So, I had the goal in my mind to fight against what the doctor told me. For three years I was up and down – my blood sugar was all over the place. Then, I realised that I *could* still eat or drink anything, I just needed to calculate the bolus dose of insulin required to compensate for the sugar content. That's when things started clicking. Not everything the doctor told me was true – I am still able to live a good life *without* all the limitations he told me about. After those first few years, there was never any question to me that diabetes could stop me and it hasn't.

When you say that you have diabetes, people tell you, 'I'm sorry.' I always reply, 'You don't need to be sorry – it's all good.' There is a lot of misinformation about diabetes.

Miguel Paludo, champion racing driver, Brazil

Any unexpected medical diagnosis is a shock, and this is certainly so for a young person who has been told they have Type 1 diabetes. One minute they are fine, running around, doing all the things that young people do, dreaming of a bright future – and the next minute, well, who knows what to think? It is inevitable that, as doctors begin to list all the things you can't now do, things will look pretty bleak. What person likes to be told, 'Stop, you can't do that'?

As someone who went through the experience myself (albeit at a very young age, so I don't remember much about the actual diagnosis), I'd like to turn this scenario on its head. I want to talk about all the things you *can* do. As you will see from all the incredible people who have contributed to this book, from sports champions to influencers to pop stars to astronauts, they've all achieved their dreams. And they've all got one important thing in common: Type 1 diabetes.

Your Diagnosis: First Steps

I was 17 when I was diagnosed and was very lucky that I wasn't hospitalised. I had lost three stone very, very quickly. And all I wanted was to drink. I was incredibly thirsty all day, all the time. I also needed to go to the toilet all the time. It was all really unpleasant. So, when I was diagnosed, it was just a relief for those symptoms to calm down. That's why I was fine with it from the beginning.

I still remember having to do my own very first injection. They just said 'hold the syringe like a dagger'. But it was fine. The only thing that upset me was the fact that I couldn't drive for a few months. Apart from that, I was just really happy to be no longer thirsty. It was the thirst that was awful.

I've never seen my diabetes as a problem and now I view it as just an integral part of who I am. It's why, when I talk to groups around the country, I'm always very keen to say, it's not your enemy. If you try to fight being diabetic, you will lose. You will absolutely lose, because you can't get rid of it. I make it my friend. I work with it and alongside it, and that's it. I think that from a mental health point of view, that's just a better way forward because it's part of me, and so I try to enjoy it as much as I can rather than anything else.

Stephen Dixon, Sky News presenter, UK

A MANUAL CAR CALLED DIABETES

If you've just been diagnosed, the first thing I would say to you is this: you *can* do anything. The key? Diligent management of your condition. The reason I have added 'first steps' to the title of this chapter is because what you do now will lay the foundation for all the amazing things you are going to do. This foundation mainly consists of figuring out your treatment (that is, your carb and insulin doses), and then you're off! In deference to racing car champion Miguel Paludo, who opened this chapter with his inspiring take on his diagnosis, let me explain my thinking through a vehicle-based analogy.

Imagine two cars.

The first car is automatic. In fact, it's one of those fancy new self-drive ones. You don't even need to steer! You get in, put on your seat belt, press a button and off it goes. It keeps to the correct speed limit, keeps an eye on

Yes, you can!

all of its own settings so it never runs out of juice and never makes a silly manoeuvre that puts its occupants in harm's way. It's got a ton of fancy diagnostics built in too, so it can fix any potential defects long before they become an issue.

The second car is a good, old-fashioned manual model. It's pretty cool, though, because there are not many of them on the road. It still goes from A to B in a perfectly smooth fashion, but the driver is in charge of starting the engine, steering it onto the highway, sticking to the speed limit and observing road hazards. Oh, and the driver needs to keep an eye on the engine, making sure it's topped up with fuel and oil and given a regular check-over to be sure it's running at its optimum level.

You and I are, of course, that cool manual model. Just as certain aspects of the car need to be controlled and maintained to keep things running smoothly, so do we. That's it. That's Type 1 in a nutshell.

> I was diagnosed in 1997, when I was 15 years old, while I was growing up in Michigan. This is the age when our bodies and life in general are changing. However, with diabetes I had to change many more things: from my study habits to my social habits. I had to start preparing a bag with pre-packed food. Back then, the treatment was a little different. Diabetics were still using syringes. There were no nice-looking pens like there are today.
>
> *Matt Collins, robotic surgery business leader, USA*

MY DIAGNOSIS

My own pre-diagnosis experience was quite typical. I was living an ordinary life and everything seemed completely fine. I was born in Budapest, Hungary. My parents were originally from villages in Siberia, Russia, but had recently moved to Budapest after deciding to broaden their horizons and that of my brother, who was 11 years older than me. Shortly thereafter, I was born. As a toddler, I was every bit as active and curious as any young child. Indeed, more so, my family say, with a slightly exasperated roll of their eyes! Then, without warning, I changed. At 3 years old, I stopped running around and became sluggish and withdrawn. I began to drink glass after glass of water, sometimes up to four litres in a single day. And I needed to pee. All the time. I even wet the bed. Feeling

Your Diagnosis: First Steps

concerned and alarmed, my parents, who were both qualified medics, took me to the hospital. I am glad that they did.

Doctors discovered that my blood sugar levels were 52 mmol/L (over 900 mg/dL). To put this into perspective, normal blood sugar ranges are between 4.0 and 5.4 mmol/L (around 70 – 100 mg/dL) before meals, and up to 7.8 mmol/L (140 mg/dL) up to two hours after eating.[1] I had, the doctors told us, the highest blood sugar levels they had ever seen. It was not a record I or my parents were happy to hold.

Initially I was broken on the day I was diagnosed at the age of 22. I lost my sense of self-identity. For the first few months, or even years, my mental health was very low. In hindsight, I'd say I was even a bit depressed. The grieving process took a while to get over. But then it all changed.

I started experimenting with a variety of different lifestyle factors and discovered solutions to the problems I was facing. I took responsibility for my health and regained control of my life and began to thrive! I can honestly say I am happier and healthier today than before I was diagnosed with diabetes. Diabetes has given me more than it has taken from me. It allowed me to discover my true purpose. It gave me a sense of direction and focus. It even gave me a new career path.

I guess you could say diabetes gave me the gift of health. Today, I'm an exercise physiologist, sport scientist, model, actor, singer-songwriter and diabetes educator – and, most importantly, I'm a happy and healthy guy thriving with Type 1 diabetes.

Drew Harrisberg, physiologist,
model and singer-songwriter, Australia

OUR DIABETES WILL NOT STOP US!

Diabetes management is not the easiest job and I won't pretend that it is. You need time to get used to it but, once you have done it for a while and got into a habit, it will no longer feel like you are 'managing something'.

---

1 'Blood sugar level ranges', Diabetes.co.uk, 15 January 2019, https://www.diabetes.co.uk/diabetes_care/blood-sugar-level-ranges.html.

Yes, you can!

It'll become part of your lifestyle, as familiar as choosing an outfit for a night out or remembering to lock your front door as you go.

Visiting your endo (endocrinologist) is also not a big deal. The appointment is not dissimilar to a trip to a hairdresser or a barber: it becomes routine. As we have seen from some of the commentators here, diagnosis is a shock at first but, given time, it can be the catalyst to drive you on to ever greater things. It could even be seen as a gift as, with time, you may start to be grateful for it. It will teach you lessons that you would not have learned in any other circumstance. Certainly, it shouldn't be something that ever holds you back. You *can* have a happy life with this condition and you *will*.

My diabetes is with me all the time. It is part of me and in everything I do. However, I do not *think* about it all the time. I think of it when I need to – when I have to make decisions about food, training, alcohol and so on. But it is not my main focus.

I got the opportunity to climb Sweden's highest mountain, Kebnekaise, thanks to my diabetes. That was life changing for me in many ways, not least because during the trip I met my best friend, who also has diabetes. Since then we have travelled together, all over the world. We've been to South Asia, Australia, New Zealand and Iceland. Our diabetes will not stop us!

Elin Sandström, health and PE student and influencer, Sweden

FIRST STEPS AFTER DIAGNOSIS

OK, you may be thinking, that is all very nice, but what is *really* happening to me?

Well, here comes the science bit, as they say. If you have diabetes, your body (more precisely, your pancreas) has a reduced ability to make insulin. Why is insulin important? Basically, it acts like a 'key' that opens doors to cells, to let glucose in to fuel your body. If that process doesn't work as it should, glucose stays trapped in your bloodstream, leading to dangerous blood sugar highs, leaving your body hungry.

Glucose is the main type of sugar in the blood. People without diabetes

Your Diagnosis: First Steps

can rely on their bodies to break down food into glucose and all the other nutrients they need, which are then absorbed into the bloodstream. Glucose levels, which rise after a meal, trigger the pancreas to make the hormone insulin, which is released into the bloodstream.

There are, as you may be aware, two sorts of diabetes: Type 1 and Type 2. We will talk more about Type 2 in the next chapter, since it can be a cause of confusion, but this book is primarily concerned with Type 1. With Type 1, your body's immune system attacks the cells in your pancreas that make insulin, so you can't produce *any* insulin at all. This means that when glucose enters your bloodstream, there's no insulin to allow it into your body's cells. So your muscles remain hungry while more and more glucose builds up in your bloodstream, giving it the consistency of, well, sugary syrup.

SYMPTOMS OF TYPE 1 DIABETES

Many people have diabetes without knowing it because its symptoms can take a little time to develop. With others, the symptoms can come on suddenly.

In the build-up stage, the symptoms you might notice include the following.

Needing to pee a lot
Our kidneys have a 'solution' to the build-up of glucose in the bloodstream: flush it out in urine. Often, one of the first symptoms is a frequent desire to pee.

Drink a lot of liquids
It might seem a bit counter-intuitive, when you keep needing to rush off to the loo, but another common symptom is a constant thirst. This is the body's response to losing so much fluid. It requires regular top-ups to keep your levels of body water normal.

Feeling tired
This is a tiredness over and above the usual lethargy felt by many young people that parents complain about. (We've got a lot going on, right?) It is a real, muscle-sapping exhaustion, where all your limbs feel like dead weights because your body can't use glucose to fuel its activities. The tank is empty.

Yes, you can!

Lose weight

One of the strange anomalies of Type 1 is that you want to eat more, but you will actually lose weight. Your body is busy breaking down muscle and stored fat in an attempt to provide fuel for its hungry cells.

YOUR ENDO AND HEALTHCARE TEAM

The foundation of a safe and happy life with Type 1 is the presence of a professional whom you trust and respect. I would like to note here the importance of having a good relationship with your doctor, healthcare team and endocrinologist. It is rare, but even today I still sometimes look at my blood glucose result and simply don't know what to do next. At moments like this it is a relief to reach out to a person who can give professional advice. If you don't like the approach of the team you've been assigned to, you can and should search for alternatives. (Definitely do not simply ignore what they say! If you ever feel like ignoring your team's advice, you are not being supervised by the right people.) Your healthcare team might not answer all your questions – after all, it's *your* body, *your* daily routines and *your* responsibility. But it's much easier figuring out the answers with their support.

I have been lucky enough to have the same doctor for the past 20 years. I see her four times a year and she has always played a crucial part in my blood glucose management. (Her name is Dr Almássy Zsuzsanna, head doctor of the Metabolic Department at Pál Heim National Institute of Paediatrics in Budapest, Hungary.) I've asked her to contribute to this book by describing the most popular treatment methods we have nowadays, so everything in this chapter was written with her close cooperation.

WHAT DOES IT ALL MEAN FOR YOU? TREATMENT OPTIONS

So, what can a newly diagnosed Type 1 patient expect today? What are the treatment options? As you might already know, you will need the following key equipment: insulin, a blood glucose monitoring device and food. I will list here the ones that I know the most about but, which version of each you go for is for you and your healthcare team to decide.

Basically, to minimise symptoms and prevent any corresponding health problems, treatment is all about control. The goal is to stay in control of your blood sugar levels and maintain them within an acceptable range.

Your Diagnosis: First Steps

How do you do this?

You need to know at all times exactly *how much* and *what kind* of fuel (food) you are taking on board. The aim is to retain a good balance between the food you eat and the amount of insulin in your body. Since you have Type 1, this means manually putting supplies of insulin into your body through injections. You need to get into a routine where you check your blood glucose levels several times a day, using a blood glucose testing device.

You need to get an accurate idea of your blood sugar levels so you can make sure everything is spot on with your insulin injections. If you add *too much* insulin into your body, your blood sugar levels will drop and you'll end up in a condition called hypoglycaemia. You'll hear this referred to with the simpler moniker 'hypo'. Symptoms of a hypo are shakiness, dizziness, sweating, headaches and hunger, and there is a danger of fainting. When this happens, to get things back on track, you need to eat something as quickly as possible.

The alternative is when you don't inject *enough* insulin (or, indeed, eat too much carbohydrate). In this case, your blood sugar goes up, resulting in a condition called hyperglycaemia. The simpler term here is 'high'. The symptoms of a blood sugar high are increased thirst, trouble concentrating, blurred vision, frequent peeing and tiredness. In this case, you urgently need more insulin, or to exercise.

The difficulty is that the amount of insulin you need to add into your body varies according to the food you eat. There are certain foods that will see your blood sugar levels soaring. (There is much more detail about this in chapter four – 'Eating Out and In'.) Other variables that will affect your blood sugar levels are sports, alcohol, illness, stress and varying hormone levels. The impact can be unpredictable, which is why you need to keep on top of your blood glucose.

I am aware that reading about hypos and highs might seem a little alarming. There is a lot of new stuff to get to grips with and understand too. It might help to give a summary of the five key things you need to stay on top of to live a happy, healthy life. They are:

- Take insulin, as prescribed.
- Eat healthy, balanced food, while keeping a careful eye on the amount of carbohydrate you consume.
- Regularly check your sugar levels by taking blood glucose measurements (self-management).

Yes, you can!

- Do physical activity.
- Go to regular check-ups with your healthcare team and make sure you receive your supplies regularly.

It's important to note that treatment is not the same as a cure. Right now, there is no cure for Type 1. You will need treatment for the rest of your life. But, as I said at the beginning of this chapter, you'll quickly get the hang of driving that manual car and will take it on some very long, happy and fruitful journeys. Yes, a diagnosis might be a shock, but you will adapt. After that, the only way is up.

THE PRIVILEGE OF HAVING TYPE 1 TODAY

The good news is that, despite there not yet being a cure, there could not be a better time to have Type 1. As Matt Collins noted earlier, when he was first diagnosed nearly 25 years ago, the options were a lot more limited. Things have changed a great deal since then and are improving all the time.

Let's take blood glucose monitoring as a case in point. When I was first diagnosed, glucose monitoring was a little hit and miss, partly because there were only so many times you could test yourself each day. Back then, the process entailed a finger-prick test to check your levels. I was always sure to do this before any significant event, whether it was presenting something on stage or taking an exam or going on a long walk. The last thing I needed was to end up with a hypo, either before or after, or worse still during, the activity. Even so, I would often find myself overcompensating, since I knew that I would not be doing another test for a while. I'd be sure to eat something with a higher carb count than usual, to guarantee that my blood glucose levels wouldn't run too low. You can guess the rest. I inevitably got it wrong and my blood glucose levels would soar. I'd then have the dual problem of the stress of presenting a talk or taking an exam, and fighting the symptoms of high blood glucose for the rest of the day.

Today, we have the benefit of continuous glucose monitoring (CGM) devices, which, as the name suggests, keep an ever-watchful eye on our glucose levels. A CGM machine is placed on your body and continuously measures the glucose in your interstitial fluid, which is the fluid in and around your body's cells. CGM is a less invasive system than finger-prick tests and works 24–7. The device has alarms that indicate when your glucose levels are too high or low. It can even be relied upon to provide this crucial information when you are asleep. Combine CGM with a detailed food and activity diary, and it is possible to make diet and lifestyle changes to vastly reduce the amount of time you spend coping with high or low blood sugar levels.

I can hardly describe how liberating this was for me. When I first got my CGM, I really felt like I was a bird, flying through the skies. The number of hypos I experienced plummeted, and everything around diabetes management was transformed into a considerably more relaxed and enjoyable process (although I'm still ever vigilant). By completely eliminating the blood glucose guessing game, I could simply wake up in the morning, go for a run and get ready for the day, all the while focused on the magnificent opportunities and challenges it offered.

At the time of writing, I have only had a CGM device for a matter of months, but I would like to add another interesting observation. Despite living with Type 1 since the age of 3, I was still largely unaware of the changes that took place in my blood sugar after I consumed particular foods. With the CGM, I discovered that they'd sometimes soar right upon eating and then go back to normal very quickly, which was completely unexpected and surprising. The most shocking revelation concerned my favourite dish, a Russian soup called borscht, which is made of beetroot, cabbage and meat. I love all soups but this one is a meal I could eat for breakfast, lunch and dinner every day, especially if it is made by my mum. It is absolutely delicious. Before my CGM, I had always believed it to be perfect for my blood glucose. It was only when I got the device that I could observe how the gauges showed an extra-fast upward pace right after I started eating the soup. I remembered that beetroot juice does indeed have a reputation for causing instantaneous spikes in blood glucose, before the insulin brings it down. Before that, I had never realised that this was the effect that the soup had. It was very informative but also sad and almost disappointing to observe.

Sad borscht moments aside, I have welcomed this new device into my life. I do, however, admit to sometimes being a bit of a perfectionist. I occasionally become a little frustrated when my blood sugar goes outside the acceptable range, particularly when I mistakenly believed I was on top of things. But, it's a nice problem to have. At least now, I always know *exactly* where I am.

Yes, you can!

Insulin

CGM is not the only development that has changed things for people like us. There have also been big changes in the delivery of insulin. These are those 'nice-looking' pens Matt referred to.

Insulin is a peptide hormone, so it will be destroyed by gastric acid if you swallow it. This means you can't take it orally, which is a shame because that would be a tidy solution. It was about 100 years ago that scientists ascertained that the best and most effective delivery method for insulin is for it to enter the body subcutaneously – in other words, into the layer of our bodies between our skin and muscle. Insulin was therefore first delivered via injection into the subcutaneous layer in 1922, not even a year after it was discovered.[2] The early syringes that were used for this purpose were pretty crude but, since they were a literal lifesaver for those with diabetes, I doubt there were many complaints. Nevertheless, they were quite time consuming to use. Made out of metal or glass, they had to be boiled in water each time to sterilise them for reuse. While a number of modifications were made in the ensuing years, including the introduction of disposable syringes, they were not ideal. Many patients (quite understandably) did not relish injecting themselves three or four times a day.

Pens

Fast forward several decades and the insulin pen arrived on the scene. Again, the pens themselves have moved on a lot since they were first used back in the eighties. Pens today are reusable and deliver a more accurate dose of insulin. They also have built-in safety features like audible clicks per dose to improve accuracy and make sure you don't deliver the same dose twice, in quick succession. Pen needles are shorter and thinner and therefore less painful. (In fact, not painful at all!) They also require less effort to inject insulin.

Technology has played a big part in recent developments, as you might expect. Newer versions have in-built calculators and record the time and date of previous injections. They can also deliver more accurate, half-unit increments of insulin. The newest developments are so-called smart pens, some of which can deliver a 0.1 unit of insulin and communicate with a smartphone application to calculate your next dose.

---

2   Rima B. Shah et al., 'Insulin delivery methods: Past, present and future', *International Journal of Pharmaceutical Investigation*, vol. 6, no. 1 (2016), 1–9.

Pumps

Another insulin-delivery development that some people prefer is the pump. The idea behind the pump is to mimic, as far as possible, the body's own natural physiology. This is where someone without Type 1 benefits from a continuous secretion of insulin from their pancreas. The pump automatically takes care of dose calculations so the amount of insulin delivered will automatically rise and fall where necessary, in line with triggers such as when and what food is eaten or exercise is taken. Sensor-augmented pumps work in conjunction with a CGM device. The newest systems can predict hypos and highs, stop insulin delivery at the proper time, or increase it if needed. The in-built algorithm predicts sugar trends and adjusts insulin doses to particular meals. It is halfway towards being an artificial pancreas.

Pen vs pumps

It is a matter of choice whether you are a pen person or a pump person. Myself, I am a pen user. This is partly because I've been using them since my childhood and they work just fine for me.

There are pros and cons of each to consider. Pumps have the advantage that you need fewer jabs, although they must be connected to a catheter (tube) placed under your skin, and the catheter must be changed every two or three days. While this process is more involved than an injection, it has the bonus of reducing the number of times you need to inject. Since pumps deliver insulin as and when needed, that flexibility is quite handy at mealtimes. If you are weighing up whether or not to have that rather nice-looking dessert, you don't need to factor in whether or not you're prepared to withstand another jab for the pleasure. The same goes for exercise. If you decide, on impulse, to throw some shapes on the dancefloor or have a kickaround in the park, you may need to take on board some carbs if you haven't adjusted your injections. With a pump, that's taken care of.

Pumps aren't all upside, though. What puts me off the most is that the pump is always on your body, since it hangs around your neck or goes in your pocket, and the needle is constantly inside you. I have never been fond of the idea of wearing such a contraption. I don't like being constantly reminded that I have diabetes, and recall feeling especially strongly about that in my younger years. Also, a pump requires attention during sports.

Yes, you can!

You may even need to take it off during some activities, which means you need to calculate how long it will be down and adjust accordingly. That all represents a lot of hassle to me and takes even more spontaneity out of life. There can be a steep learning curve for the first few weeks of pump use (although that is not necessarily a big deal at a time when *everything* to do with Type 1 is pretty new). The cost can be prohibitive too. There is also a risk of skin infections from having a catheter implanted under your skin. Plus, there can be issues with getting air in the tubing or blockages, which will mean that you won't get enough insulin.

If you would like a doctor's viewpoint, I will share what Dr Almássy believes, which is that a pump is the way of delivering insulin that is most physiologically similar to what happens naturally in the body in people without Type 1. She says that if you are ready to compromise by having a pump on your body almost all of the time, it makes your life easier and healthier.

After noting all of these points, I will say it is entirely your choice. There are many people who manage very well with pumps and love them, and, equally, the same goes for pen fans. It's a question of lifestyle and personal preferences. I would never stop anyone from getting a pump. It is an amazing piece of technology and works wonders for some people.

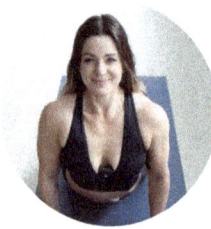

My pump wire gets caught on the kitchen doorknob every day. I start walking away and then I can't walk anymore – I just laugh. I'm stuck. That's pretty funny. You just have to laugh at yourself about that.

Evan Soroka, yoga therapist, USA

THE FUTURE FOR TYPE 1S

Things continue to change and get better when it comes to treatment and management for Type 1s. Most recently, there have been trials of something very close to a true 'artificial pancreas'. The system uses algorithms to automatically adjust insulin doses throughout the day and night. It is early days, but initial results suggest that this could be another big step forward in making the management of diabetes much easier and more precise. The message is: watch this space.

Despite all the advances, I know that you will become overwhelmed after your diagnosis. It happens to everyone, and you should expect that. There will be days when you'll just be completely fed up with thinking about the food you're eating, or the activities you are taking, or what the hell is going on with your hormone levels. Don't worry – that frustration is completely normal. But, think about it in another way: there are frustrations with day-to-day life whether or not you have Type 1. Things don't go as expected, plans go awry, or you have to really focus on something that needs to be done that maybe you don't particularly want to do. Managing Type 1 is just another one of those things that needs to be looked after as part of your day-to-day life.

2
TELLING OTHERS

Yes, you can!

One of the worst things to happen to me was when a business partner in the music industry told me not to tell anyone that I had diabetes. He believed that it would ruin my career and lead to organisers being unwilling to invite me to concerts. I became genuinely scared that I would not be able to do any more performances. It instilled a real fear in me to even admit I had diabetes. I was troubled about it too. It was absolutely not how I was raised. My mum always taught me to be completely honest.

After one year of this, I stopped working with this person and I decided to openly admit that I have diabetes. Ever since then, I have been very open about my condition. It was really interesting to see what happened then, because immediately people started coming to me. Now, whenever someone in Russia is diagnosed with diabetes, I am one of the first people they look for. I think doctors say to patients, 'Don't panic! Famous people like Kornelia Mango also have diabetes.' After that, the first thing newly diagnosed guys do is reach out to me. I get DMs in Instagram saying, 'Kornelia! I have diabetes! What should I do?'

It is very important not to hide your diabetes and not to hide yourself. If you do, it will be much harder to explain later on in the relationship with your partner, your friends and your colleagues.

Kornelia Mango, singer and celebrity, Russia

Once you have your treatment sorted, you may be thinking, OK, now how do I show myself to others? There is a short answer to this and it is the same as before: be yourself. You are always the person who sets the tone when talking about diabetes.

OPENING UP

There was a time when people were very secretive about Type 1. This was particularly so for teenagers, who are naturally very keen to fit in and just be thought of as one of the guys. It's not a nice feeling to stand out as someone who is 'different' in some way, even if it is because of something you have no power to change. My view is that this situation has changed a lot, even in my lifetime. This is probably due to a combination of factors, with one of the most significant being social media. We're a lot more used to being open about things (even if it is from behind the safety of a keyboard) and the internet is, as Kornelia Mango's experience shows, a great place to find some answers to all of the questions that buzz around in your head when you're first diagnosed.

My parents recently admitted to me that the year I got diagnosed, they decided to make it their main task to help me see diabetes as very natural. Part of this 'campaign' was that my mum always injected me in public. I certainly remember that they were always easy with taking out our own food in restaurants and were very open about it with their friends. They definitely invested a lot of energy in my diabetes and as much in my perception of it as in the management of it. They never wanted me to hide in the toilet. Instead, they encouraged me to explain proudly why I do what I do whenever someone enquired. Whenever my dad saw me being hesitant to eat or inject in public, we would have this simple conversation:

Dad: 'Why do you hide yourself?'

13-year-old Kristina: 'I'm afraid they will think badly of me.'

Dad: 'So what? It's their problem. Why are you worrying about strangers' problems?'

They believed that if I treated my Type 1 casually, everyone around me would do the same. Now I'm older, I can see how right they were. No one ever really thought badly of me and I certainly never, ever experienced a hateful reaction.

When I recently asked some of my friends and relatives to tell me what stories they associate with me and diabetes, they reacted like they had been given an impossible question. Most of them had a hard time even remembering any and, after a couple of days of me badgering them to remember *something*, the answers were almost all the same.

'I never really associated you with diabetes. It has never defined you, and certainly never was an obstacle in our relationship.'

Most of the diabetics I know have a similar experience with those who are close to them.

THE REVEAL

But, I am getting ahead of myself. What is the best way to broach telling people around you that you have Type 1? It may not always feel all that easy to slip into conversation, especially if you are just getting used to the subject yourself.

The average age of diagnosis of Type 1 is 13,[3] and the ease of how and when to tell others may vary according to where your own diagnosis falls around this metric. Your condition might well be something that you don't feel ready and willing to discuss with your crowd. I will do my best to tackle the various scenarios here.

Telling others that I have diabetes was never a huge issue for me. As detailed earlier, I was diagnosed at a young age (3 years). This means I've never really known life without diabetes. It has just always been there. I grew up with diabetes by my side. I have no memory of ever being able to eat whatever I like, whenever I like, without having to think how much insulin I'd need to inject. Therefore, I have no regrets and nothing to compare my life to. Likewise, I have become accustomed to going with the flow and mentioning Type 1 at any convenient point as I get to know people. It just seems like another cool fact about me. I certainly don't remember consciously contemplating developing a specific technique to inform people. It has always been a very easy and natural thing to bring up, whether it is on the first, or tenth, meeting with any new acquaintance.

It might be helpful to go into a little bit more detail about my own experiences and the reactions I received from others at each stage of my upbringing. I can't guarantee it'll be the same for you, but I suspect there will be a lot of similarities, especially if you were also diagnosed at a young age.

KINDERGARTEN

Kindergarten was, without a doubt, the most straightforward stage. Young kids really don't notice the differences between them. I am also very grateful to my mum for carefully selecting my kindergarten. She chose a place where absolutely healthy kids were mixed with ones who had particular medical needs. There were kids there with diabetes, food allergies, lactose intolerance and gluten sensitivity. We were all supervised by trained nurses, who made a wonderful job of not only taking care of us but also making sure that we were all absolutely normal and healthy

---

3 'Understanding the extremely early onset of Type 1 diabetes', Diabetes.co.uk, 2017, https://www.diabetes.org.uk/research/our-research-projects/south-west/understanding-the-extremely-early-onset-of-type-1-diabetes.

kids. This ensured that I spent my childhood in an inclusive environment, playing with the rest of the group. No one ever laughed at me or mocked me because I was 'different'. This helped to build a firm foundation where I understood I had nothing to be ashamed of. (Which, of course, we don't!) I truly wish every child who has a condition that requires attention could have the same experience and be looked at as an absolutely normal kid from the earliest stages.

Looking back at that time now with a more analytical eye, my abiding memory is that we were *all* very different, but also very similar. We were just small, noisy human beings, starting out on our individual adventures to explore the world. We all wordlessly accepted our various conditions as *just as things were*. When we got a bit bigger and the others who didn't have any conditions began to notice, very little was said. By this stage, I had completely recovered all of my pre-diabetes energy and athleticism, so I could chase anyone who dared laugh at me.

PRIMARY SCHOOL AND HIGH SCHOOL

While I still wasn't absolutely responsible for my actions at primary school age, my mum did a great job of helping me to find my own way. She made sure that the school's management, teachers and catering staff all knew I had diabetes. But they never really had to do anything with this information, apart from ignoring the times when I brought out food to treat a low during a class. Really, that was it. Aside from this intervention, my mum left it up to me to decide who I shared my condition with. I never really felt mocked at primary school. Diabetes was so natural to me that kids couldn't help but accept it.

Later, I switched to an English-speaking high school where nobody knew me. I was a bit more independent by this stage and did not welcome my parents going in to speak on my behalf. However, this meant I had to tell all my teachers myself. Unfortunately, I had almost zero skills in English back then and, well, perhaps the message got lost in translation. This was completely down to me. I hated the English word 'diabetes' and preferred the literal translation from the Hungarian word *cukorbeteg*, or 'sugar sickness'.

Despite my early awkward linguistics, I felt it a duty to explain to people in charge why I behaved the way I occasionally did and, most importantly, why I needed to eat during lessons or exams. One of the most interesting moments was when one of my teachers replied to my big reveal with a 'Hey, me too!' He became my go-to person whenever I had to share something, or needed something, with regard to my 'sugar sickness'.

My life changed hugely after being diagnosed. I was 19 years of age and it just came out of the blue. It was completely unexpected. With Type 1, there's no 'easing in' to living with the condition. You're thrown straight in at the deep end. I remember getting a call from my doctor, very early in the morning, and him telling me, 'Your blood tests came back. You're diabetic.' My blood glucose levels were dangerously high and I was rushed into hospital. It's strange how something that I really didn't know anything about was immediately my daily priority and has to be for the rest of my life.

I've never had an issue with telling people I'm diabetic. If you're diabetic, you should be confident and proud about it. The fact that you're living with it each day already shows people that you're no push-over.

Each time people discover I'm diabetic, or see me using my supplies, I get a similar reaction. Typically, it runs along the lines of, 'You're diabetic?! But you're not fat! Is it because you ate too much sugar? My grandad is diabetic. I deeeeeeeefinitely couldn't inject myself every day!' And so on. I've also had a few odd looks over the years while injecting in public. I've seen some offended and disgusted faces. If you don't like it, don't look. Simple as that!

Eoin Costelloe, personal trainer and model, Ireland

BECOMING A TEENAGER

You will note that I have spoken a lot about the advantages of being diagnosed very early on, because obviously this is the scenario I know the most about. Those diagnosed at a very young age have a different experience from those who get a diagnosis in their teens. While I am sure it is quite disruptive at the time if you are diagnosed as a youngster, most of that disruption is borne by your carers. I do, however, think that I experienced at least a little of what someone might feel if they are diagnosed in their teen years in my own teenagerhood. Certainly, this period was a big turning point for me.

The teenage years are ones of major transformation for everyone. We start making friends, going out, dealing with problems and enjoying our time *independently*. Often that comes in a form of rebellion, but the point is to make decisions ourselves, even if those decisions are very, very wrong. I definitely associate this period with starting to make my independent choices around blood glucose treatment.

Up until this point I had been following the very rigid instructions of my parents and my doctors. I was an exemplar kid (overly so, maybe) so the thought of going beyond any instructions didn't even cross my mind. Then, those sweet teenage moments arrived and I started making treatment decisions. I reckoned that I was fine and could manage very well. However, the pendulum had swung very quickly from being bound by rules to freestyle decision-making. The way I started 'breaking bad' was with my own personal drug of choice: food.

It would be easy to blame my crowd. (Why did they prefer fast-food places?) Ultimately, though, it was always my choice. I had never been deprived of any particular foods because I had always done loads of physical activity. This means that I wasn't rebelling against food itself. I was just proving to myself that I could make food and treatment decisions on my own, without my parents. You know – my body, my life, my business. Needless to say, once I started experimenting, my blood sugar rocketed up to somewhere in the upper stratosphere. It was definitely a rocky period health-wise. It did seem a little unfair, though. The biggest concern of other teenagers was to decide which movie to watch, or how to get home after a good hangout with friends. My biggest concern was making sure my mum didn't find out I had high blood glucose. Again.

Finally, after my regular three-month check-up revealed an all-time, record high average blood glucose, it took a lot of willpower to get myself back on track. The solution was just going back to the routine from which I'd been so desperately trying to break free. Even so, there were definitely a few, quite silly, 'wilderness years' that I now regret. But then again, what teenager doesn't say that whether or not they have Type 1?

There were some periods as a teenager when I was a little scared that I wouldn't fit in, make friends and be part of the 'in' crowd. But these thoughts were quickly erased as soon I found myself in the middle of a huge, family-like teenage friend circle. I had friends, loads of them. They were always very, very understanding about my condition. Ultimately, the only way I was different back then was the same way I am now: I need to be more careful about what I consume. But, happily, life can be enjoyed in so many other ways!

If you are diagnosed as a teenager, I'd imagine (and fully understand!) that it might seem unfair to have diabetes at such a time. Yet, trust me, in the long term it is really a trait that makes you more independent and much more mature than anyone else in your friend circle.

My advice to anyone is to be open about it and even to show off. When a new friend says 'Wow, you are so disciplined' or 'Wow, you do so much sport' or 'Wow, your eating habits are so on point', this is when I show off the secret behind my superpower.

'Yes!' I will reply. 'That's because I have had diabetes since I was 3 years old. It helped me develop this skill.'

After that, no one ever answers with 'Ah, I am sorry.' It always encourages them to learn more, to listen and to understand more about the condition, with all its upsides and downsides. In fact, as a teen, I played this scenario for so long that some of my friends began to say, 'Yeah, doing sports is easy for you – that's your gift from diabetes.'

I went through a phase in my teenage years when I made it my job to hide my diabetes from people I met. I never wanted to be seen as weak, different or not worthy of love. Everything shifted when I started to understand that the world sees you how *you* see you. And that's when my journey to self-love and embracing my Type 1 began.

Lauren Bongiorno, diabetes health coach, USA

INSULIN INJECTIONS

Another big issue in my teen years was insulin injections. Until that point, I'd been entirely comfortable about the place where I topped up on insulin. I did it because I had to. It never felt awkward at kindergarten or primary school, because everyone knew me and had grown up alongside me and my condition. I have always been very natural with my injections and still am today. I've always known it is an essential part of my wellbeing, so I have tried to make sure others perceive it in a similar way. I do notice people feeling uncomfortable when I inject. They might stop their conversation, ask what I am doing or simply pretend they didn't see anything. If you've never seen an insulin injection or done one yourself, let me just briefly digress to explain. The pen or needle is injected into the hand, stomach or legs and needs to be held in place for around ten seconds or so. This ten seconds can feel like a very long time indeed when you are in unfamiliar company, and people often can't help but give you curious looks.

Occasionally, strangers will even feel duty bound to butt in and moralise. 'It's not appropriate to do drugs in public places!' is a phrase anyone with Type 1 will be familiar with. My opinion is that everyone's reaction is their own business. Meanwhile, I am minding my own business, which is staying healthy and strong no matter the circumstances.

I remember a number of years back, myself and a group of friends went on a trip to Spain. A close friend of mine had always been terrified of needles (soft, I know). It was the year I had been diagnosed, so he obviously was around needles more often. He said, 'Eoin, I wanna get over my fear of needles.'

Long story short, I poked a tiny, empty needle in him. He was pleasantly surprised that it didn't hurt or even look as bad as he had anticipated it to be. He was delighted that he had 'overcome his fear of needles'. So, I struck again and dabbed another tiny, tiiiiiiny needle in him. Again, he barely even noticed and was happy to claim he had beaten his fear.

A few moments passed, then he took another look down at the two needles in his abdominal area, went as white as a ghost, passed out and fell headfirst through a window!

Everything was fine in the end, although he's now even more terrified of needles.

Eoin Costelloe, personal trainer and model, Ireland

It took me a little while to work out my own personal strategy for dealing with the stares and potentially negative comments I experienced from new acquaintances. However, I did get there in the end. Firstly, I realised that when I ate where I wasn't supposed to, or injected in public, it would always provoke comments or odd looks. There was no use hiding it or feeling embarrassed. This is just me: get used to it.

Secondly, I drew upon my upbringing, which was very open and honest, and decided that this was actually an *opportunity*. I needed to stop worrying about what others thought of me and turn their curiosity around. This was the perfect time to inform and educate others about Type 1, so they understood why I do what I do. Hopefully they'd be more understanding the next time they saw someone injecting themselves with insulin.

Thirdly, I decided I needed to relax into my role and have some fun. I let the mischievous side of my personality come to the fore. With time, it becomes enjoyable to start eating an apple in a place where you are not supposed to, such as a bar or nightclub. Or, even better, to chew it loudly in the middle of an exam. No one is going to stop you! I've learned to rather enjoy the surprised looks I get when I pull out a chocolate bar in a restaurant and eat it to treat an urgent low, just as everyone is digging in to their starter. For some, these actions might seem unusual, but the people who truly matter to you will always understand. My friends always laugh (in a nice way) when I do these things and they always look forward to the next crazy move.

Today, I am very comfortable talking about my diabetes. In the beginning, though, I would hide it because I hadn't yet identified with it. I felt embarrassed and ashamed. If I was out in public, I'd go to the restrooms to test my blood sugar and inject insulin. However, after years of living with it, I am now fully transparent when it comes to managing my condition. I'm proud of the way I manage it. I want to be a spokesperson to inspire and empower other people to accept their diabetes and use it to fuel personal growth and development. I like to call myself an authentic, transparent guy, so it only makes sense to be open about my diabetes because it is a part of me and my story.

I find most people are intrigued. They'll ask what I'm doing when I'm pricking my finger or injecting insulin, but it's nearly always out of curiosity, not judgement. Well, that's how I perceive it anyway. It seems like not many people are familiar with it.

Drew Harrisberg, physiologist, model and singer-songwriter, Australia

PEOPLE GET CURIOUS, ABOUT DIABETES AND ABOUT YOU

What would my advice be about telling others if, say, you are a teenager who has just been diagnosed? Of course, the decision is very personal and it is up to you, but I would say: don't feel you need to hide it. Diabetes is just another cool trait of your unique personality.

When you tell others that you have diabetes, remember that they will perceive it in exactly the same way as you do. If you announce it with worry and self-pity, people around you will think about it that way too. In contrast, if you say you've got Type 1 with your head confidently held high, it will not be discussed negatively in any way. Think of it like a fashion model starting a new trend. At first their style might be mocked, because it is different. However, when they confidently and happily continue to show off their uniqueness, the once unusual trait becomes an enviable feature. Discussing diabetes in a positive way (as your superpower) helps you embrace it, own it and turn it into your friend.

Reactions will vary from person to person. Some people will be very keen to talk about it and ask loads of questions because they are really curious. A lot of people with Type 1 talk about others asking to 'have a go' with their blood-testing kits. They'll want to watch the injections, or talk about what you can and can't do. Some of my best friends and colleagues have been so curious about my condition that they've gone on to learn everything about it from scratch. This is all great. Spread the word. The more people who know, the better. You'll also find that they're very willing to help. If you say you need a snack or a coke, they'll be the first to get up to go and get you one.

Another good thing about people knowing about your Type 1 is that they can look out for you. Those close to you will immediately notice if something is not quite right and will always be supportive if you aren't feeling 100 per cent. Once, one of my friends (not diabetic) sacrificed the last piece of her favourite doughnut because my blood glucose was low. Imagine that. She had been talking and dreaming about the 'limited edition, five-star-review doughnut' for a month. Yes, there is such a thing.

Yes, you can!

The place it was sold from was very far outside London and my friendship group eventually agreed to make it our weekend hangout programme to visit the doughnut shop. We bought my doughnut-loving friend the last one available for takeaway. But guess whose blood glucose decided to sink low on the way home? She almost had tears in her eyes as she asked me if I needed the doughnut and went visibly pale as I screamed, 'Yes!' I ate her cherished piece of food but didn't leave this huge gesture unnoticed. The next time I visited her, I arrived with four identical doughnuts to express my gratitude: it was a happiness overdose! Kindness like this means a lot to me and I am proud to have many friends (and I know you have them too!) who are so selfless when it comes to treating my lows and highs.

Just as there will be those who are curious about every detail, there will be some who barely acknowledge it at all when you tell them you have Type 1. They just won't see it as a big deal. But that doesn't mean they won't jump in if you need assistance. This is great too. Even if they don't know exactly what to do, at least they'll notice if you are behaving oddly, which might indicate a looming emergency, and will be primed to call for an ambulance if necessary. This is the main reason why I personally prefer telling people about my condition. I've never had a situation when my blood sugar has become so low that I couldn't treat it myself. However, my close friends know the hypo routine very well, should anything happen.

If I ever (very rarely) encounter someone who thinks I can do less because I have diabetes, or sees me as an incomplete person just because of the condition, then I know straight away that this is not a person with whom I wish to interact for any period of time. You're free to make your own judgements on this one. Maybe I am just not very tolerant!

Another useful tip is not to be tempted to gloss over things. If my interaction with someone new develops to a stage where I need to refuse the offer of a piece of chocolate or a cookie because I don't feel like eating it, or spending energy on adjusting my insulin to accommodate it, I am very careful about what I say. My refusal is always polite but never dismissive. I am sure to explain that I have diabetes. It is much better to outline the background to the refusal, rather than saying a blunt 'no' to a friendly gesture or being oddly vague about the reason for your refusal. When you turn a kind offer down, people can easily feel offended. If you give a (brief) explanation, the person offering the treat will understand much better and it may well spark the next topic of conversation.

STRANGER WITH TYPE 1? HELLO, MY NEW FRIEND

Whenever you spot another person with Type 1, you have an almost guaranteed friendship! Diabetes makes it unusually easy to connect to others who have it too, or who are good friends with someone who does.

Whenever I meet someone else with Type 1, it often feels like I've just encountered a long-lost sibling. After five minutes of interaction with this somehow familiar stranger, you will be in awe of just how much you have in common. These moments remind me how wonderful our community is.

I remember one time when I was a student attending an event at my university. It was quite early on and I didn't know anyone. I deliberately chose a seat in the same corner of the lecture theatre as a group who seemed quite friendly, or certainly pretty lively. To begin with, we didn't interact much. We were too busy listening to the main speaker, who was naturally the highlight of the event. Then, during the break, I noticed that one of the members of the group was checking his blood sugar. All of his friends clearly knew what he was doing and all their attention was glued to the meter measuring his blood glucose. I noticed that everybody was completely silent and even seemed to be holding their breath in the excitement. I smiled, because I've seen this before in groups of friends with a Type 1 among them. Everybody is wondering: what will the result be?! When the monitor stopped beeping and the results were revealed, everybody started high-fiving the guy. They were all whooping and saying 'Well done!' and 'Awesome!' That's when I thought, 'This is my moment to make new friends!' I waited until everybody had calmed down and then I literally started staring at them (who says I didn't go to uni with some amazing social skills!). Then I grabbed the sleeve of my jumper and waited until everyone noticed that I was staring at them all. When the final person looked at me, I pulled up the sleeve, and *voila!* I proudly showed off the CGM on my arm. The reaction was something like that of a football team when they score a goal. We all started high-fiving each other. I was inundated with questions and in an instant it was as if we'd known one another for years. Later on, we ended up going out to dinner together and I am still in close relationships with this amazing group. They are all great examples of fantastic friends who truly care about the lives of people around them. Look out for people like this. There are plenty of them around us.

Yes, you can!

CONFUSING TYPE 1 AND TYPE 2

There's still that stereotype that there's just *one* form of diabetes, which is Type 2. A lot of people come up to me and say they know stuff about diabetes. However, they are talking about Type 2. They'll say, 'Oh, my grandparents have Type 2 diabetes.' Or they'll explain that their parents check their blood sugar every morning. It's clear they're talking about Type 2.

What I want to push for is more recognition of the *difference* between Type 1 and Type 2. I feel like it's my duty to be a voice for the Type 1 community. In order to teach people about this difference, someone like me only needs to put in a little more work. When I check my blood sugar or use my insulin pump and somebody asks me a question about it, I take it as an opportunity to educate them and let them know that there is a difference between Type 1 and Type 2. I explain that I have Type 1 and then tell them more about what is required from a person living with this disease.

It's just a matter of breaking down that stereotype and leaving that person with the knowledge that there is a difference. I show them that what they once thought has changed. It means they are more aware of this disease and I hope that's helpful for the next person they encounter living with diabetes.

David Mina, graphic designer, USA

Ask anyone with Type 1 about their experiences of telling others about their condition and they will almost certainly tell you that it is often confused with Type 2. Type 2 is the most common form of diabetes, accounting for around 90 to 95 percent of cases according to the Centers for Disease Control and Prevention in the USA.[4] Thus, if people know anything about the condition at all, they're far more likely to know about Type 2, or even know someone who has it. But the two conditions are, in fact, different.

---

4 'Type 2 diabetes', *Centers for Disease Control and Prevention*, 30 May 2019, https://www.cdc.gov/diabetes/basics/type2.html.

Telling Others

I've already talked you through Type 1, but, for clarity, when someone has Type 2, it means their pancreas still produces insulin. However, thanks to insulin resistance, the body is unable to use it properly. The cells become less sensitive to insulin, which makes insulin less effective at lowering blood sugar.

While both forms of diabetes can be down to genetics – if you have a family history of either condition there is more likelihood that you'll get it – there is another factor that comes into play with Type 2: lifestyle. Obesity and physical inactivity both contribute to the risk of developing Type 2 because they make it a lot harder for insulin to do what it is supposed to do. Therefore, while there is no known way to prevent someone from developing Type 1, adjusting your lifestyle and diet, and being more active, can prevent or delay Type 2.

Type 2 is also a progressive disease that might well worsen over time. As a result, the pancreas needs to work harder, needing to produce more and more insulin to overcome resistance. Eventually, the insulin-producing cells 'burn out' and insulin production stops. Thus, some people in the later stages of Type 2 need to take insulin.

Another key difference between the two conditions is that Type 1 is usually diagnosed in children and young adults, whereas its counterpart is generally diagnosed after the age of 40. This is changing a little, alongside the childhood obesity epidemic, so we are seeing more young people with Type 2, which is another reason the two conditions are easily confused. The treatments are very different too. People with Type 2 may be prescribed oral medicines in the early days, although, as indicated here, they may need insulin as the condition progresses. Lifestyle changes are also crucial.

> I think people have an element of sympathy, or understanding, certainly in the UK. But, I do think there is generally more education required. The only thing that gets annoying is that there is obviously a big issue with obesity and Type 2 diabetes in younger people. So, you still get this confusion with people thinking that we're to blame for having Type 1 because of our diet or lifestyle. I always try to refer to myself as Type 1 now, rather than just being 'diabetic', as a result of that. Generally, though, I find people are absolutely fine about it.
>
> *Stephen Dixon, Sky News presenter, UK*

Yes, you can!

There are a *few* similarities. The conditions share similar symptoms, such as excessive thirst, increased need to pee, unexplained weight loss, tiredness and blurred vision. Plus, of course, Type 1 and Type 2 both need to be carefully managed.

If you have Type 1, you had better get used to a certain amount of confusion and misunderstanding. Unfortunately, there will be a lot of people who will associate you with their parents, or grandparents, or overweight friends or relatives. Occasionally, when you tell people you have diabetes, they will think you are joking. They'll say, 'But you are the last person who will ever have it, because you eat well/do a lot of sports/ etc.' When this happens, stay calm. When people try to show their knowledge about the topic (even if the knowledge is not quite right), they are trying to connect with us. Just reply, 'But diabetes is one of the main reasons why we eat well/play sports/etc.' It can be frustrating, but the best way to look at it is, it doesn't matter if you are Type 1 or Type 2. They are both diabetes. The conditions are similar to each other and there really is no point getting offended if there is any confusion. Say thanks for the person's interest, explain the difference if you wish and take the initiative to spread awareness about Type 1.

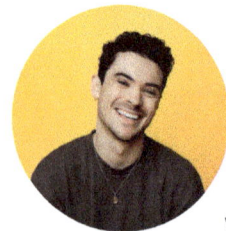

People look at me and go, 'You're diabetic, but you're not fat!' It happens all the time. People don't really understand. There are over 4 million people in the UK with either Type 1 or Type 2 diabetes, and only 10 per cent of those have Type 1. So, it is easy to feel like we're in this isolated community.

Fortunately, we are actually the most proactive community, because we didn't choose this condition or bring it upon ourselves. We want to change it, do something about it and cure it. This isn't always the case with Type 2, where you can make your situation worse in certain cases. They're completely different conditions.

I'm really working hard to change attitudes towards Type 1. I use whatever platform that I have to educate people about what Type 1 is. The more people that understand it the better – not least, because if you have a hypo and people know that you're diabetic, they'll know how to deal with it. You want

> people around you that know what they're doing.
>
> Jonny Labey, actor, UK

TELLING OTHERS HELPS

For anyone who is likely to have some sort of relationship with us for the medium to long term – whether at school, university or work, or just a general friendship or a more personal basis – it is fair to let them know we have diabetes. Why? Because sooner or later you might get in a situation where it is your diabetes talking, not you. At these times, it is a good idea to make sure people speak your language. They can be on hand to help if you do start to feel ill. People around you also need to be alert to the potential 'side effects' that come with this special group of people with Type 1 (by that I mean the occasional 'crazy' behaviour I referred to earlier, such as eating in unconventional places!).

It's really up to you how much you share or tell anyone. You can, if you wish, keep explanations short and sweet, tell people that you have to eat certain things and inject at certain times, and leave it there. Remember, though, you should feel no embarrassment about having diabetes.

Let me leave you with one final thought in this chapter. This concerns the power of having amazing people around you. There are times when diabetes can be a hard thing to handle, especially psychologically. If you don't have it, it is hard for others to understand what all this 'insulin–carbohydrate' balancing really means. Some will dismiss it as eating and injecting and that is it. But it's not that straightforward. Far from it. At times a blood glucose chart follows a very curvy line, despite all the effort put into balancing everything. While we can still absolutely live well and be very happy indeed, achieving as many great things as any other person in this world, it can just become a little too overwhelming sometimes. Type 1 can occasionally feel a little like a full-time job from which you can't even take a holiday. Mentally it is always there, locked into our heads. If you don't stay focused, you can suffer bouts of unhappiness, despair or even depression.

The worst possible thing to do is to suffer in silence, or refuse to discuss your fears and anxieties with others. Therefore, it is great to have people around, not only for emergencies (when they can step in and help) but also just to be there emotionally if ever you feel overwhelmed. I truly value my absolutely wonderful friends and family, who are there with me

Yes, you can!

at the breakfast, lunch and dinner table, helping me decide how much to inject, because they have come to know my patterns. Even though they can't understand exactly *how I feel* when I'm not at my best, they know *what actions to take* to maximise the chances of me being well. They can help me to make decisions when I simply feel tired of it all. My fantastic friends always seem to choose the right words to give me power when I need it because everything has become too much and I can't help but cry out 'Maaan, why?!' One of my friends in particular is a very good motivator and supportively says, 'Kris, hold on, you are so, so strong. You can do everything and even more than this.'

Understanding and cheering words from people whom you admire and trust, and who believe in you, can truly make a ground-breaking difference in the quality of our diabetes management.

3
CONFIDENCE

Yes, you can!

I have always lived by the maxim 'the future belongs to those who believe in the beauty of their dreams'. I had always dreamed about climbing Everest or being an astronaut. When I was diagnosed with Type 1 at the age of 24, I was told to forget about those dreams. 'A diabetic has never succeeded in these endeavours,' I was told. I was in shock for several months. I had no idea about diabetes or what it was. Then, I learned, diabetes is just a travel companion!

Everything changed radically for me. I had to learn how to eat and train differently. I wanted to push myself to the limits. I kept thinking: if other people can do it, why can't I? And I did. I did the Seven Summits, which is an international project that involves climbing the highest mountain on each continent. I was the 288th person to do this and the first with diabetes. Then, I went on to convert the Seven Summits into a Grand Slam, which additionally involves dragging a sled weighing 125 kg to both the North and South Poles. That was tough. They took two weeks each, but I reached the Poles without any help.

In the past few years, I have been living at NASA and training in the Yuri Gagarin Research and Test Cosmonaut Space Centre. The physical training has been really tough. I can't use diabetes as 'an excuse'. There are no excuses: either you are well prepared or you are not. Eleven times I've been in a centrifuge, which exerts a G-force (G) of 5.4, where your head weighs 80 kg and each arm weighs 48 kg. We need to withstand a weight that is eight times normal. If you move even a millimetre, you can break your spine and be paralysed. I've also trained in the hydro-lab, in a one-to-one scale replica of the International Space Station, carrying out exercises in a space suit weighing 135 kg. And I have piloted a MiG-29, the most advanced fighter plane in the world.

I have already done a stratospheric flight, but am in training to go into outer space as the first ever diabetic astronaut. During training, these machines don't know if I am diabetic or not. I need to do the same manoeuvres as everyone else, in

Confidence

> search of 4 or 5 Gs, so my body knows how to respond when we go into space. There are *no excuses*.
>
> Josu Feijoo, mountaineer and astronaut, Basque Country

Whatever you like to do, diabetes is not an obstacle or an excuse. It is, as Josu mentioned, a companion. For some it is a travelling companion, for others it is a co-pilot, while for others it is a dancing partner. Our confident life with diabetes starts by including it in our everyday activities. Just what kind of companion you turn diabetes into depends on the life you choose to lead.

YOU CAN DO ANYTHING WITH DIABETES

If you ever find yourself saying, 'I can't do that because of diabetes,' *stop right there*. You can do anything you want to do. You really can.

Positive mental attitude is important. Yes, there will be challenges, but that doesn't mean you can't overcome them. Throughout this book, there are stories of people with Type 1 who have done some truly remarkable things. In moments of contemplation, I often wonder: would they have done these things if they hadn't been diagnosed with the condition? Yes, I'm pretty sure that they would have. They are all driven and dynamic individuals. But, did their diagnosis drive them even harder, so they could *prove* themselves just that bit more? Or, and this is another possibility, did they just decide to make the most of every single day? Certainly, living life to the very fullest has another added bonus. When you pursue an interesting and varied life, your attention is constantly occupied by what you are doing. It's only when you are bored that the doubts and anxieties have space to creep in. So: get busy.

> The TV show that I took part in was called *I Can*. It was a very engaging show where each week we had to learn a new skill, such as jumping on a trampoline and doing a back or front flip, learning to do beatbox rap and learning how to play a traditional Russian Harp. I love dancing, I love singing and my performance wasn't affected by diabetes in any way! This is a lifestyle and by now, for me, it is automatic to manage it around whatever I'm doing on a daily basis. Diabetes is not so scary when it is being taken

care of. If you accept it, make it your friend and turn it into a lifestyle, then your life becomes much more manageable.

Kornelia Mango, singer and celebrity, Russia

CONQUERING THE WORLD OF FASHION

Diabetes has been a companion to me in many different ways and throughout numerous activities. In this chapter, I will describe two experiences that left significant marks on my life, boosted my confidence and proved that I can, indeed, realise my dreams. I am aware that they are not extraordinary achievements at all compared to some of the unbelievable successes of the participants of this book. But they are moments that illustrate that we can still notice and enjoy every detail of this life with diabetes by our side.

Being diagnosed very young meant that I had a lot of time to think about what I wanted to be when I grew up and, yes, I admit there was a part of me that wanted to prove to the world that I could be something pretty special. I wasn't going to be held back by Type 1 and there was absolutely no reason that I should be. For me, there was only ever going to be one choice of career. For as long as I can remember, I wanted to be a fashion designer. No, that is not quite correct. I wanted to be a *world-renowned* fashion designer!

I can still remember the look on my parents' faces when I announced, at the age of 15, that I was going to attend the best fashion university in the world. Although they both looked proud and clearly admired my ambition, they couldn't disguise their underlying feelings of doubt and concern. Why? Well, in my view, the best fashion uni in the world is Central Saint Martins, which is based in the centre of London. Not only was it in a different country, but it was also slap bang in the middle of one of the busiest, most thriving cities in the world. How would their daughter manage in a strange country, with all her special dietary and lifestyle needs?

To their credit, they gave their guarded approval. I suspect they realised that their headstrong daughter had made up her mind and was going to doggedly pursue this dream anyhow.

Armed with their consent and my own excitement, I threw myself into doing whatever I thought it would take to realise my dream. Nothing was going to hold me back and certainly not my Type 1. I instigated the switch from the Russian school I'd been attending to join an English-speaking international school. I reasoned that a sound grounding in the English language was essential. Outside school, I signed up to regular drawing classes and went six times a week. Over time, I trained my once horrific pencil-management skills into what I would now proudly call 'decent artistic skills'. For five years, the wonderful, crumbling, damp-smelling drawing studio hidden deep inside Budapest city centre, where I took these classes, became my own cosy little space. If I had any spare time, I would spend hour upon hour leafing through fashion magazines. I was hungry to boost my knowledge, understanding and flair for the subject and was not going to waste a moment. I really couldn't wait to get to London.

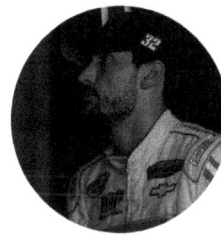

While racing in NASCAR, I was named by the International Diabetes Federation as one of their Blue Circle Champions. Since then, I have tried to spread the word about diabetes as much as I can, showing by example that *diabetes can't and will never stop me*.

Miguel Paludo, champion racing driver, Brazil

In early 2016, I heard about Regent's University's 'Wearable Architecture' competition. Regent's University, which is also based in London, was launching this annual contest to create a single item of clothing, or a collection, based on an architectural theme. It would, the entry brief advised, be great if entrants kept up with fashion by checking out magazines and websites, were aware of all types of designer, and were ready to draw and design with imagination. *This contest was designed for me!*

It was as though everything had come together and was pointing to this one event. London was my dream city to visit! This fashion design competition was, literally, my ticket to London. If only I could get shortlisted, I could visit and see the city of my dreams. I can barely describe how engaged and excited I was, but my blood glucose readings clearly reflected it; they were perfect in this period. Mind you, I was so determined that I had no other choice but to make sure I was in control of my blood glucose.

The next few months were a whirlwind of activity as I worked on my entry. I must have gone through dozens of themes as I tried to settle upon one that would catch the eye of the Regent's University judges. I eventually decided to focus on the theme of 'stairs' – specifically, a spiral staircase – and designed a collection of asymmetrical dresses. I enlisted the help of a very able dressmaker, who was able to translate my somewhat ambitious ideas into a rather impressive 3D structure. To finish the spiral staircase effect, I adapted some shoes, as well as a bracelet, so they mimicked my unique pattern to complete the look.

It wasn't until my entry was complete and submitted that I really had time to draw breath and think properly about it. And then I was very nervous indeed. It felt like submitting a lottery ticket, the prize of which was visiting London and observing my design on the catwalk. I was up against people from all over the world who had trained in art and fashion design. It was a tall order to even expect a place as a runner up, let alone to win. Yet, visiting the city was my dream and I was so close to making it come true.

Then, at last, I received news from Regent's University. Unbelievably, against all the odds, I had been shortlisted! I was one of just three on the shortlist.

I didn't really think of it at the time, but looking back there was a certain satisfaction that I'd proved to myself that diabetes was never going to be an obstacle. As long as I kept my management of it on track, I really could do whatever I set my mind to.

Some weeks later, I was off to London. And then, just when I thought my life couldn't get any better, it did. I won! I could barely believe it when they announced my name. It was, without a doubt, the happiest moment of my life to date. It was when I finally truly believed I could do anything I wanted. And what a feeling that was.

I was 13 years old when I was diagnosed and realised that I needed to be more aware of what was going on in my life, because everything changes when you get diagnosed. You have to just think about your life and what you can do and what you need to take extra care with. Even though I was given a manual on diabetes and instructions, there is so much else that you learn by trial and error. Even though I was a teenager, I knew I had to be very mature and listen to my body. It took me a long time to understand that I had to put diabetes first and not push it aside. You really have to just make a huge shift.

I think discipline takes a long time to develop. Well, it took me a long time to become disciplined. You need to develop self-awareness to see the correlation of your patterns. It is possible to get habituated to our patterns. We get used to how we're eating, or how we're administering insulin, and then sometimes we just get stuck. We don't see that what we're doing is not working any more. It takes practice to get used to and that's why I'm a yoga practitioner. It helps me create space for myself on a daily basis, to get quiet and observe not only diabetes but also my whole life. I then reflect on what I can be doing differently. What's working? What can I change? What can I let go of? That kind of stuff.

Evan Soroka, yoga therapist, USA

TYPE 1 FOR CONFIDENCE

Your diagnosis will improve your life. Yes, it really will. Why? Because you are now adopting a lifestyle that is all about self-discipline, self-awareness, willpower and healthy activities. As Josu Feijoo so rightly says: there are no excuses.

Self-confidence and self-belief don't happen by accident. They are not things that you are born with (although I accept that some people do seem to have more confidence than others). True confidence comes from a lot of practice and many small successes, which over time build into larger successes. If you have a goal, commit to it, continue with your good habits and management of your Type 1, and your confidence will start to grow. And so will your successes. The more you familiarise yourself with your body and its reaction to the treatment, the more confident you will become in living life monitoring your blood glucose.

There is a large element of 'fake it until you make it' when it comes to confidence. It's very easy to shrink away and think, that's it, I *can't* do all the things I want to do. It doesn't help that Type 1s are often told by well-meaning people in the medical profession that they might need to reduce their expectations once they have been diagnosed. I can't help but notice that this is a common theme among many of the people interviewed for this book. Yet, as so many have proved so far, Type 1 is rarely an excuse. My

Yes, you can!

way of dealing with anyone who is in the least bit negative about what I might achieve is to turn their view on its head. Let it fuel your ambition and drive to succeed, no matter what. If there is an important event coming up that will lead you closer to your goal – whether it is an interview, a competition or meeting someone new – dress for the part, hold your head high and show them just how amazing you are. Your inner confidence will make you come across really well. What's more, you will feel great and a lot more confident about what you might be able to achieve.

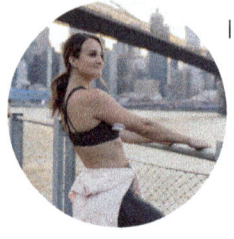

I attribute much of my resilience and drive to having diabetes. I face challenges multiple times a day, so not much outside of my diabetes seems impossible when I'm constantly priming myself on how to overcome these day-to-day hurdles.

Lauren Bongiorno, diabetes health coach, USA

Always appreciate the positives in your life. It's easy to let negativity slip in (especially if others are telling you to temper your expectations) but that doesn't help you achieve a happy life with diabetes. Take a moment to look at all the great things you can do, whether it is drawing well, running quickly or understanding complex mathematical equations. Focus on how much better your life is because of what you can do. If you practise this sort of single-minded positivity in your daily activities, you'll eliminate any room for negativity. You'll realise things are a lot better than you think they are and it will equip you with the wherewithal to achieve your goals.

You can't ignore Type 1. There is clearly much to be done in managing it. However, go one step further than 'merely' managing it. Accept it and realise you are perfect the way you are. Do your very best with the hand you've been dealt: you will be amazed at what you can achieve. As long as you get started, you will make progress.

Confidence

> The main focus of my life is to continue to create opportunities for myself and my family to be successful and leverage that success to help our communities and our neighbours to do the most good – whether that is advocating for people with diabetes, coming up with creative advertising solutions or travelling around the world with the people I love.
> Life is a confidence game, and when you have confidence in yourself things tend to work out for you.
>
> *Rob Howe, entrepreneur and founder, USA*

The great thing about building your confidence is: it will stand you in good stead if anything doesn't quite go as you wanted. And remember, things don't always go to plan whether or not you have Type 1. To illustrate this, let me finish my story about my ambitions to take over the world of high fashion.

EXPECTATION VS REALITY

Following the competition, I earned my much-coveted place at Central Saint Martins. I was so excited about it that I completely ignored any warnings from my friends in Budapest. Those who claimed to know a little about London and the fashion scene made ominous predictions about what I might find in the English capital, most specifically the uni. It's one of the toughest educational establishments in the world, I was told. It's hugely competitive and students are so desperate to excel they barely get any rest. It is not unusual for design students to be slaving over projects 24–7. And, my friends warned, the rivalry is intense.

Nonsense, I thought, dismissing their concerns as, at best, misinformation and, at worst, jealousy. Sure, lack of sleep and stress can play havoc with our blood sugar, but hey, there is no way it can be that bad, right? Plus, I had managed a pretty demanding schedule thus far. How difficult could it be?

Well, my friends' prediction turned out to be quite accurate. If you have ever seen the movie *The Devil Wears Prada*, it might give you a bit of an idea about what a cut-throat, ruthless business the fashion industry is. In fact, for a while I joked that the film must be a documentary! When I started at Central Saint Martins, I embarked on a six-month foundation course, known as Fashion Folio. The idea was to follow it up with a three-year BA course. I gave the foundation my all. I really did. I worked harder than I had ever worked before in my whole life (put together!) and stressed myself out more than I had ever known. While I learned more about one subject and myself than I had learned throughout 13 years at school, I realised fairly quickly that this was not the life for me. It was nothing to do with managing my diabetes – it was more to do with the fact that this way of working and viewing the world did not suit my values. I was not being judgemental, because it was a great course and there were plenty of people who thrived on it; however, it was just not for me.

Let me tell you now, it takes a whole heap of confidence to say, actually, guys, I was wrong. This world-famous fashion course I have been banging on about for so long? Yeah, well, about that. Turns out it wasn't the right thing for me after all.

Just like with anything, when you try something for the first time, sometimes you fail, other times you succeed. Either way, you'll have learned a valuable lesson for next time. Even though I am not doing fashion, or even drawing on a consistent basis any more, the experience taught me to learn things step by step. Painting in the beginning was very, very hard. I had no idea what I was doing. With time, I managed to complete a decent painting at least ten times faster and better than before. As I became more confident, I knew where I needed to add colour and how to draw shapes. It's the same with diabetes. It might seem like loads of work in the beginning, but with time you will make much better, more effective and almost automatic treatment decisions.

> Diabetes is just one cog in the machine. In saying that, diabetes is a full-time job. I am always testing my blood sugar and administering insulin, but that doesn't mean it rules me. I've learned to love it and manage it so that it doesn't manage me. I've reached the point where my control is relatively effortless. It's as if I'm on autopilot.
>
> Drew Harrisberg, physiologist, model and singer-songwriter, Australia

BUILDING CONNFIDENCE

I had a big decision to make. Go back to Hungary with my tail between my legs, or press on and realise my dreams of success, albeit in an entirely different discipline from fashion. The going-home option was immediately dismissed from my mind. I had tasted the freedom and energy of London and there was no turning back. However, my biggest challenge was that my A level results were not exactly stellar. With just a few years to learn English *and* pass challenging exams in the language, my grades had not been good.

It was at this point that I pressed the pause button and had a good think about what I really wanted to achieve. I didn't want to start another course with gusto and then drop out disillusioned several months later. After much thought, I decided that I would pursue a career in business. I hadn't liked the fashion course, but I had very much enjoyed the free-thinking, creative side, and in particular the idea of starting my own label. Some sort of business course would be the best way to channel my entrepreneurial energy.

After a few false starts, I was accepted onto a half-year foundation course at Queen Mary University of London, which I finished with a distinction. This opened a lot more doors for me and after weighing up my (expanded) options, I opted to continue my studies at the Cass Business School (also in London), embarking on a BSc Business Management with Digital Innovation and Entrepreneurship course.

> My dreams have changed a lot since I was younger. I was always very active and involved with various activities and sports. I put myself under pressure because I was good at a lot of things, but struggled to pick one to really go for. I had dreams of being a professional skateboarder, footballer or artist. Sometimes I didn't know what it was I wanted, but I knew I wanted to do something big and be the best at whatever that was.
>
> *Eoin Costelloe, personal trainer and model, Ireland*

I realised almost as soon as I started at Cass that I had made the right decision. I loved the course and it reflected my own beliefs and aspirations. I felt really motivated and inspired. That is not to say that I never made a mistake or a mis-call ever again. Ironically in a chapter about confidence, my biggest mistake at this time came via a business called Connfidence.

Yes, you can!

I'll tell you about it to show that, even when you know 100 per cent what you want to do, there will be hiccups along the way and almost all of the time they will have nothing whatsoever to do with your Type 1.

My colleagues at Cass were all from different backgrounds, but what unified us all was a lot of ideas about amazing businesses we would run. Inspired by the hot-bed of creativity, I followed in the footsteps of many of my fellow students and started my own business as a sideline as I completed my course. It was something we were all very much encouraged to do, not least because practical experience is invaluable while studying business. Naturally, most of us were drawn to the possibilities of ecommerce, as this seemed like the most appropriate way to run an entrepreneurial venture while also studying full time.

So far so good. Move over, Jeff Bezos: the next big thing is on the way! After exploring various ideas, I decided that drop-shipping was the answer. For those not schooled in the world of business, drop-shipping is a supply chain management system where an entrepreneur doesn't actually physically keep the goods in stock that they are selling. They're more of a middleman (or woman), passing their customers' orders to manufacturers or wholesalers, handling the money, and then leaving it to the manufacturer or wholesaler to actually dispatch the goods to the customer. Easy, huh?

And the product I decided to build my would-be drop-shipping empire around? *Roll of drums*: earrings! I found a supplier in China and made an agreement with them, and produced a tidy little website. Such was my conviction that I was 100 per cent onto a winner, I called the venture Connfidence.

Now, if you have any sort of business background at all, you might be giggling a little now. The shipping costs from China were disproportionately high when compared to the low cost of the earrings. And then there was the very real marketing flaw in that earrings are often an impulse buy, yet my customers would have to wait weeks and weeks for them. Needless to say, over six months I sold just *six* pairs of earrings. I chalked that one down to experience and closed Connfidence. Fortunately, it did not dent my own confidence too much. It was just another experience on my path to better things and I learned a lot along the way.

Confidence

Your diabetes – your own damn rules. It will take time to know what rules and routines to put in place to make you feel as good as possible, and these may change over the years. But don't forget that life is changing and that your routines need to be adjusted as well. You will become a professional and best at knowing your own body and your diabetes. You decide.

Sara Mobäck, influencer, Sweden

WE ARE AWESOME

Despite the ups and downs of my early career, my view of the possibilities open to me have not wavered. I am still hugely optimistic about the future and relentlessly positive about what I can achieve. (You will read more about my current endeavours in the later chapters.) The idea of pursuing our dreams is an important lesson for us all. When you are leading an interesting life, your attention is occupied by all that you are doing. It is only when you shy away from doing things, or lack the confidence to try something, that you withdraw. The worst outcome then is that you will become bored. Boredom is a terrible thing for anyone, but I feel it is even worse for a diabetic. It gives your worries space to take over your mind. For us, that main worry is the ups and downs of our blood glucose. It is inevitable that in such circumstances, you will overcompensate, or try to fix something that's not broken. (I did not think of my blood glucose levels once during the six-month period of Connfidence and ended up with record good measures, so that's something!) So: don't let yourself get bored. Dream big and don't let diabetes discourage you: have it by your side, get up, get out and take on the world. You are awesome!

4

EATING OUT AND IN

Yes, you can!

> I don't eat healthily just for diabetes; I eat healthily as just a human. If I wasn't a diabetic in the next life, I'd choose to eat healthily because I want to feel good. I want to feel strong. I want to live long. That's the beautiful incentive that I always push to everyone else. Eating well is for a bigger, better reason than just hitting our blood sugar numbers.
>
> *Ali Abdulkareem, blogger and job coach, USA*

Let me clarify right from the beginning. *We can eat everything*, but we need to dose well with insulin to make sure the food doesn't spike our blood sugar. There is no given food that we can't eat… *however*, if we return to the superhero vision in the introduction for a moment, we do have a weak point. You could think of it as something like Superman's kryptonite. Our kryptonite is any food that has a carb count we don't know about. Therefore, our weak point is any food where we have to guesstimate our insulin injections.

> Food is your friend. It is vital for your body to be functional. Don't listen too much to all the tips and advice on different types of diets or dietary advice; it can confuse more than it actually helps. Food should be and is joy and you can eat just about anything if that is what you want, even if you have to think a little bit more about the amount of food or insulin. For example, it's better to have a little candy now and then, rather than to eat the whole thing all at once on Saturday night.
>
> *Sara Mobäck, influencer, Sweden*

UNFAMILIAR (EATING) ENVIRONMENTS

Eating well wasn't a real challenge for me in the early years of Type 1. I barely even thought about it, to be honest. My parents kept a close eye on my diet and made sure I had a healthy and balanced range of food. They helped me to understand what my food routine should look like. My mum put a lot of effort into researching the amount of carbs in individual dishes and in ingredients. Later on, when I began looking after myself, I knew exactly what each dish was made of and how many carbs there were in them. My friends called me 'the food scanner', because I could always tell them what they had on their plates.

Things changed a lot for me when I moved to London at the age of 18 to take up my coveted place at Central Saint Martins. I wasn't just leaving my home, in the city where I had grown up; I was also going to live independently for the first time. Plus, I knew precisely no one in London. When I first arrived, all I had was me, my suitcase full of clothes and an empty room – and, just to add a bit more to the sense of anxious anticipation, I had to grapple with the added bonus of a cold with a high fever. Meanwhile, I didn't know the city at all, so I had no idea of the appropriate places to buy food or, if I chose to dine out, where to eat. Even though my carb knowledge was good, and I felt safe, I realised early on that adapting to local food would be much trickier than I thought. This was the moment that I found out that Indian vegetable curry, Japanese teriyaki chicken, and Chinese sweet-and-sour dishes are not as carb free as they sound. In fact, they were almost worse than desserts. For my entire life beforehand, I'd been used to eating very transparent food. Russian and Hungarian cuisines are quite straightforward: proteins and some carbs and veggies – perfect for a diabetic. It was pretty easy to track carbs. London, however, introduced me to food cultures from all over the world. I quickly realised I had to step up my 'carb count' game.

Having never really looked at the detail of the ingredients and preparation methods of foreign cuisines, I felt a little vulnerable. How would I choose the most appropriate meals? In a big city full of every type of food possible, there could potentially be multiple hidden dangers. Hidden carbs are everywhere! It took some time to learn what's what, but, through trial and error, I now have confidence that I could, if I wanted, eat those meals with much less guesswork.

My Type 1 was discovered during a routine health inspection when I got a new job. I was 28 years old and they caught it right at the beginning. It was obvious from the start that no drastic changes in lifestyle were required and I can live quite freely as a diabetic, too. Early on, I tried to keep to scheduled meals and eat at specified times, but I've abandoned that since then and I don't worry much when I eat at a different time or skip a meal.

Yes, you can!

> I'm sure that my meals have gotten more regular recently, though, and wherever I go, I do think about what and when I'm going to eat that doesn't have (too much) sugar but enough carbohydrates so that my blood sugar level doesn't drop. Also, my alcohol consumption changed in that I almost never drink cocktails or liquors, only dry wine spritzers.
>
> *Csilla Németh, influencer, blogger and photographer, Hungary*

EAT ANYTHING, BUT KNOW WHAT YOU EAT

Anyone with Type 1 will know that there's a lot to get to grips with and food is one of the very first things we need to understand. You will notice that I am very deliberately not saying 'restrict'. I don't think we should say 'no' to our favourite treats. However, we do need to become familiar with what we eat. Most importantly, we need to become familiar with carb counts. Yet, it is not something to panic about.

In the past, it was the norm for people like us to be given a fairly restrictive diet plan. This was because insulin was not as freely available as it is now and treatments were more restrictive. Treatments today are far more flexible, insulin works more quickly than ever and the monitoring of blood sugar levels is much more accurate. All of these developments combined mean we don't have to worry so much about a long list of restrictive dos and don'ts. In fact, when it comes to what you can eat, the recommendation is largely the same as that for everyone, regardless of whether or not they have diabetes: eat a wholesome and balanced diet.

You will need advice and training from your healthcare team to help you understand how to manage the amount of carbohydrate you eat versus the quantity of insulin you need, so you can effectively control your own blood glucose levels. It may seem like a bit of a faff to begin with, but you'll quickly learn your body's insulin–carbohydrate relationship. This is something that is very personal to you (which is why you need advice). To give you a small example of how important it is to 'know yourself', even if my diabetic friend and I are ordering the same meal in the same restaurant, we always inject different doses in order to end up with similar blood glucose levels. We are all different. We're different sizes, with different body requirements and different daily routines.

Consistency and discipline are key. In chapter two, I mentioned going off the rails in my teen years when I rebelled with what felt like the greatest contraband of them all: fast food. I became highly influenced by the less-than-healthy food habits of my friends. Fast-food restaurants were our go-to place (affordable and tasty – what else do young people need?). No one even considered healthy alternatives. Not surprisingly, my once carefully managed blood sugar levels turned into a chaotic roller coaster ride. After all, even when you know how much to inject, fast-food is not a type of food that keeps blood glucose stable if eaten every day. Oh, and despite still doing a lot of sports, I also put on 10 kg. Quite a teen rebellion, huh? Fortunately, I worked out how much damage I was doing before it became a real issue. I still eat fast food sometimes, if I fancy it, but only rarely. And, when I do, it is always in a much more disciplined manner.

Nowadays, whenever I find myself eating out in the middle of the working week or socially, my meal choice is usually based on food where I am familiar with the carb count. Occasionally, though, if I go somewhere purely for the pleasure of tasting some new good food with my friends, I have to do my best to guess. Sometimes it works and sometimes it doesn't. When it does, it is one of the most satisfying feelings ever. When it doesn't, it's no problem. I view it as a good lesson and resolve that, next time, I'll estimate better.

I usually cook for myself each day. I find it a lot easier to keep my blood levels within a healthy range it I know exactly what's going into my food and how much. It can be difficult eating out sometimes, because you don't necessarily know the amount of sugar (carbs) that are in your dish. Most of the time you will find yourself guessing the amount of insulin you will need. This can lead to inconvenient and unexpected highs or lows.

More often than not, if I'm out for food, I will order something with a very low carb count, like a salad. Most of the time my need to keep my bloods level is a lot more important than me indulging in sugary or high-carb meals. Saying that, though, I'm only human, so of course there are times I say 'f*** it' and treat myself to a portion of sweet potato fries so big it could feed a small village.

I always say that if I wasn't diabetic I'd be twice the size.

Yes, you can!

> I would be eating Chinese food a lot more frequently. There's never a time when I wouldn't want to eat it. Sweet and sour chicken balls, fried rice, curry sauce on chips... I can almost feel myself drooling as I say this. My brothers and I used to do everything in our power to try and convince our parents to get Chinese food for dinner (before I was diagnosed). Now I need to convince myself *not* to get it!
>
> I love food and have a serious appetite. Sometimes it's difficult to be strict with my diet for the sake of my diabetes, but I know how important it is.
>
> *Eoin Costelloe, personal trainer and model, Ireland*

ROUTINE HELPS, BUT WHO CAN STICK TO ONE?

I certainly agree with Eoin regarding his note on portion sizes. And the thought that your blood glucose might go off track if you eat certain foods definitely boosts your willpower and motivates you to plan your food in advance. The big problem with planning is, well, who has a consistent life? Something that my transition to independent life showed me was that it is very easy to get thrown off track in terms of diet. From the start at Central Saint Martins and then at Cass, my schedule was quite hectic: running from a team meeting to a lecture, making sure I was prepared for presentations and projects (on time), and ensuring I met all agreed deadlines. I am never one to shy away from long hours, and this can make things quite difficult when trying to eat regular, nutritious and balanced meals. Fortunately, my continuous glucose monitoring (CGM) device takes a lot of the guesswork out of things by making life a little bit more predictable even in unpredictable situations, but it is not always ideal. Nevertheless, planning your meals in advance can certainly make blood glucose management more seamless and less demanding of your focus throughout the day. Meal planning might not only mean pre-cooking your own food but also going to dining places where you are very familiar with the carb count of the dishes on the menu. If there is a day when I don't have time to prepare food for myself in the morning, I'll visit a place where I already know how my blood glucose will react to the food. However, cooking and calculating your own food is always the surest and most consistent approach.

Eating Out And In

> Sometimes you will just want to have a dessert and there's nothing stopping you from having it. The only difficulty is knowing how much carbs is in it, because looks can sometimes be quite deceiving. Say you're having a sticky toffee pudding. You'd think the sugar is all in the glaze, but there's also a lot of sugar within the sponge. There's always little things like that, where you underestimate how much sugar is in it. It is a lot easier these days with continuous blood glucose monitoring.
>
> *Jonny Labey, actor, UK*

Another potentially tricky situation is any sort of event, whether it is a presentation, meeting new people or networking. You don't want to be in the position of getting into a low or finding yourself in a high right in the midst of a significant discussion. It's happened to me a few times and I am not fond of these moments. I know full well that at times like this my main focus instantly shifts from the person (or the topic) to my blood sugar and forces me to think of ways to improve my blood glucose in the moment. My best advice is to avoid these roller coasters and make sure you follow your routine diet, but to take extra care. I've learned to eat properly before important events and to always check my blood glucose beforehand. This way, I can be sure to direct all my attention to the event in question.

> I feel the biggest challenge for anyone who has any special dietary requirement is to know as much as possible about the said condition, allergy or requirement. I know from my own experience that learning about diabetes in my personal time has made a massive difference and been of exceptional benefit. Being aware of what you can and can't eat is crucial in your day-to-day living.
>
> *Eoin Costelloe, personal trainer and model, Ireland*

LONG-TERM DIET PLAN

On a day-to-day basis, there are a few rules that you will need to follow to create and maintain a good, long-term diet plan. Your medical team will take you through their own recommendations and it is wise to follow them. They will most likely discuss the importance of good carbohydrates (vegetables, pulses, wholegrains) and the difference between fast carbs (sugar drops, sugary drinks, some fruits) and slow carbs (oats, beans, mixed-grain breads). Make sure you pay attention to your doctors and do your research about your favourite foods, to make sure you are fully aware of the carb counts of your routine meals.

You might notice that there is a market in foods labelled as 'diabetic' or 'suitable for diabetics'. Naturally, they come at a premium. The general advice is to avoid them: if you want an occasional treat, go for something you really like and just keep an eye on your portion sizes.

Something else to think about is sugary drinks, which can be good and bad. They make your blood glucose levels shoot up very quickly, which is a really handy treatment for a hypo, but they can be difficult to manage if you are just drinking them on a day-to-day basis. It is, however, good to have one to hand. To show how handy they can be, let me give you another example of something that happened to me.

The incident occurred when I was 16 years old and still back in Budapest. It was a cold, grey winter's morning and, for reasons I can't quite recall, I decided to take a long walk before starting my drawing class at 9am. I realised fairly quickly that I had not dressed appropriately for the weather conditions, since it was bitterly cold. I felt pretty uncomfortable by 15 minutes into the walk. My fingers and toes felt like blocks of ice, my nose was dripping and my eyes stung with the effects of the cold wind. Worse still, I was dizzy. The obvious reaction required was to immediately check my blood glucose. However, this was not an enticing prospect. I didn't have my CGM back then, so the process would have involved pricking my finger. The thought of taking my already frozen hands out of their place deep inside my pockets was a non-starter in my mind. Besides, I had checked my blood glucose before I set out, so it wasn't that, right?

I trudged on for another ten minutes, feeling progressively colder and out of sorts. By now, I was shaking too. Then, I realised that I had begun to sweat as well, which seemed crazy in the intense cold. There was no doubt in my mind: something was not right.

I looked around me, searching for a warm café where I could take refuge, check my blood glucose and get myself sorted. Of course, it was 8am on a weekend morning and everything was shut. There was nothing for it: I sank down on a nearby bench and wrenched my hands out of my pockets into the freezing air. It wasn't easy to do my usual checks, but when I did, I was shocked. I was rocking 1.8 mmol/L (30 mg/dL). Given that I usually start feeling the effects of a low at 4 mmol/L (72 mg/dL), this was very worrying indeed. I was quickly losing my senses now. Fortunately, I always carry a bottle of sugary juice with me, so I downed it in one go. Then, all I could do was to wait for it to kick in. It was a hugely uncomfortable few minutes. I was sitting alone, out in the cold, early in the morning, shaking and barely conscious. I was with it enough to notice a few stares from passers-by who clearly thought I had had too much to drink. I don't blame them for their judgement – how were they to know? It was a pretty painful episode, though.

What lessons did I learn from this? First and foremost, always carry a sugary drink with you. Secondly, never hesitate to check your blood glucose if you feel the least bit weird. And finally, when your mum scolds you for not dressing according to the weather, don't ignore her!

> I just try to eat really well-balanced meals, but I count everything. I have an app and I just put it all in. I follow macros so there are certain percentages of fat, carbohydrate and protein.
>
> While I try to stay balanced with my diet, I do really believe in the saying that everything should be in moderation.
>
> *Evan Soroka, yoga therapist, USA*

LEARNED YOUR ROUTINE AT HOME? IT'S NOW TIME TO STEP UP YOUR GAME!

Something that anyone with Type 1 will get to know quite quickly is that there is a world of difference between eating in and eating out. It is very easy to get into a routine at home and become very familiar with the carb and sugar counts in all your favourite dishes. There are, however, two issues we can't control when we go out: the people who work in the restaurant and the menu on offer.

I will start with the first point. One of the biggest issues when eating out is that serving staff don't always really 'get it'. While most people understand peanut allergies or gluten intolerance, they often come unstuck when it comes to carbohydrates. Or, carb counts can be confused with calorie counting. Questions about the menu will elicit curious responses about whether or not the diner is dieting for weight-loss purposes. This can often be followed by the 'helpful' offer of a salad, which is only slightly ruined by the accompaniment of a sickly, highly sweetened dressing, such as sweet chilli or Thousand Island. A serving of these dressings often contains at least four tablespoons of sugar. Er, thanks but no thanks, guys!

We need to be on constant alert to make sure that our servers register the seriousness of our requests. Please don't misunderstand my motivations here; we don't need to explain to anyone *why* we order what we do, but sometimes sharing your condition with the staff of a restaurant ensures they take any requests seriously.

Once, when out with friends in a bar, I ordered a drink with a diet coke mixer. While the barman was busy mixing, I double-checked with him to make sure that the coke that he'd added was indeed of the diet variety. He nodded, but there was something about his nod that unsettled me. It was absent-minded and appeared to be just a little uncertain. So, I pressed the issue. I explained that I had diabetes and if the coke was not a diet one, I would have health consequences. I told him that if this happened, he would be entirely to blame. The result? The barman took the drink away from me, poured it down the sink and made a new one.

My advice: be brave! Let bar and restaurant staff know your requirements, and never be shy to press the point home.

You also need to work with your server to get an idea on the timings of serving. I have had experiences of being told that my food would arrive in 15 minutes, which means I inject to make sure I can eat as soon as the food arrives. Then, after waiting 30 minutes (!), I get told 'sorry, another 15–20 minutes'. This is when I know that I have to treat my blood glucose urgently and start cursing myself for not making it clearer to the waiter that I have diabetes. If you prefer to stay unnoticed, the easiest thing to do is to order a juice to keep yourself safe. However, the number one rule is to always have food with you, even when you go to a restaurant, so you can make sure that your blood glucose will not drop, even if the food is delayed. Today, I always specify in advance that I need the food on time because I have Type 1 diabetes, and it always, without exception, arrives on time.

And so to point two – the menu. When you eat out, it's difficult to predict precisely what you'll get. While you may well be familiar with many of the dishes in question and may even have cooked something similar at home, the challenge is that you have no idea how much of any sugar, oils or other ingredients has been added to make the dishes more flavoursome. If you don't know, it becomes very difficult to administer the appropriate insulin dose. If your best guestimate is very wrong, it can have a significant impact on your blood glucose levels. Other dishes, which you maybe wouldn't usually have at home, will often have a huge amount of hidden carbs. Think here of rich, sugary sauces, or syrups in coffee.

My advice is to check the menu of the place where you wish to go beforehand. If it seems really complicated, choose somewhere where it is more straightforward so you will be able to have at least a credible guess at how many carbs there are in the meals offered. Once you are seated, don't be afraid to discuss with the waiters what is in the meals you are about to order. It is not unreasonable to ask them to double-check with the chefs about the details of certain ingredients. This will make it easier for you to determine how much insulin to inject.

You may be a little reticent to ask all these questions, or feel that you'll seem like a fussy eater. Let me tell you this: you won't be the first person who has asked a waiter to double-check something. I once spent some time working in a very busy restaurant that served fine French cuisine and I feel like I have seen and heard it all! I was asked on a daily basis what was in the dishes. There was a variety of reasons given, from gluten to dairy to egg intolerances, or specific diets, whether vegan, vegetarian, keto, pescatarian or paleo – the list goes on! Some days it seemed like every single person needed to make sure that a certain ingredient was not present in their meal. I got a lot of exercise running back and forth to the kitchen to check. The best cases were when people brought their own food in a lunchbox and handed it over to us with the instruction to 'heat it, put it on a plate and decorate it as if it were the restaurant's offering'. (By the way, this is also an alternative you can follow. If your family or friends wish to go out to a place where you know that you'll struggle to find anything carb-predictable, just bring your own!) Of course, we had to do it, because we were trained to value our customers and follow their requests, especially when these were related to dietary requirements. It was also the best thing for these particular people, as it gave them peace of mind about what they were eating.

It is in a restaurant's best interests to make sure you are having a great experience at their establishment. It will result in your positive feedback and, most probably, see you want to return. So, go on – don't be shy. Bomb your waiters with questions! They are very much used to it.

> In the past few years there has been a huge wave of people with diabetes sharing their journeys on social media. We all have voices and the more we continue to share our stories, the more diabetes will be understood. In terms of food overall, in the USA there are certain states, such as New York and California, where healthy food is more accessible. Further afield, there have definitely been improvements, with many more places offering gluten-free options or even some blood-sugar-friendly options on their menus.
>
> I really love when restaurant menus are labelled with 'GF', 'DF' or 'V' (gluten free, dairy free or vegan) because it makes the process of deciding what I want a lot more enjoyable! I believe in empowering the customer, whether that's on packaged foods or in menus, so they ultimately can decide what will work best for them and not have to rely on guessing or be misinformed.
>
> *Lauren Bongiorno, diabetes health coach, USA*

As Lauren says, things are improving all the time when it comes to the variety on offer for those with differing requirements. As I noted when recalling my brief waitressing career, there has been a marked shift towards more health-conscious and environmentally aware eating. The hospitality business now offers a far wider range of food options on its standard menus to cater for different demands. Purely and simply, these are commercial decisions for restaurants. Many restaurants are also becoming far more transparent about the food they serve. It is not unusual to find nutritional facts and ingredients laid out on menus. I should probably add that in some menus, this is still confined to a special section of 'healthy options', which will feature a handful of dishes with predictable carb counts. Still, things are heading in the right direction.

Bear in mind that if you end up eating something that you are not familiar with, or have any doubts whatsoever, simply check your sugars a bit more often and take action whenever you see something not going well. It is all about the timing and as long as you catch any ups or downs on time, you will be able to enjoy your dining-out experience. Once again, never be afraid to check your blood sugars or to do injections in public. Deciding to miss out on things just because you are afraid of others' opinions is a sure path to unstable blood sugar levels and an unpleasant eating-out experience that is memorable for all the wrong reasons.

In some restaurants, they display how many calories there are in the foods. Other restaurants are advanced enough to write out the carbohydrates in their foods. If it was this way everywhere, dining out would become much easier. Otherwise, sometimes you find yourself really wanting something, but you'll be very scared. In those moments I usually choose to eat meat (such as a good steak) and some vegetables.

If each restaurant provided exact information on the ingredients they had in the meals they offered, *or* simply indicated how many carbs there are, our lives would become much easier because then we could calculate the insulin that we have to inject in order to feel good.

Kornelia Mango, singer and celebrity, Russia

HELLO, NEW DINING EXPERIENCE

Earlier, I mentioned my move to Cass Business School, to embark on a BSc Business Management with Digital Innovation and Entrepreneurship course. There was, as you may recall, the false start with the earrings venture. After I realised that was going nowhere, I was left to reflect on what other entrepreneurial venture it might be helpful to cut my teeth on. It's always good to work on something you are passionate about, which is why my next venture was in the field of eating out – more specifically, in restaurant foods that suit a particular diet.

My thought process went something like this: there are so many food trends nowadays, eating out while trying to stick to a specific dietary lifestyle is not always easy. Wouldn't it be great to build a platform that makes this easy for customers? The key was to find a way for restaurants to complete orders in a more flexible way.

Yes, you can!

The business idea I came up with is a service app that helps you tell restaurants the recipe of the dish you want so they can cook it for you. It's not unlike having a personal chef in any restaurant you go to. The app is also handy if you don't know how your food is cooked. My team and I have built the app in such a way that you can order dishes prepared using the recipes of the people you follow (be it your doctor, a favourite food blogger or a chef) in the dining establishments you visit. The business, which I called E77, helps dining outlets adapt to each customer's order. (Feel free to visit our website: www.e77.io.)

Once I had gathered a team that could help me develop the service, the idea was endorsed by Cass's incubation space, the City Launch Lab. It's been through a three-month accelerator programme, where I've learned some crucial skills on how to grow a venture like this. Now, despite some rough critiques and a series of sleepless nights, we have the E77 app ready to download and use, with restaurants that wish to use it and customers who are excited to be served personalised meals. E77 is the venture that, so far (and to my own surprise), I have been the most proud of. We've been given grants, successfully developed the product for mobile and web platforms, and been nominated for the Business Innovation of the Year 2019 award by the Restaurant & Takeaway Expo – and our journey has only just started! E77 has also helped me to realise that I love what I do. I am constantly seeking ways to grow. I hope to spread this service widely, to make dining out easy for people with various dietary requests.

The lesson I have learned here is that persistence pays off, whether it is in your professional or personal life. Watch this space, as they say.

> The biggest challenge is always when you are in a situation where you can't decide what to eat. This usually occurs when you're with a group, or at an event where either the choices are limited or the need of the community determines what those choices are. It's often hard when you can't eat something that everyone eats, because it's easy to feel like you are losing out on something.
>
> Csilla Németh, influencer, blogger and photographer, Hungary

The message from everyone I spoke to for this book is that life is getting easier for Type 1s when it comes to eating out. Many ambitious young entrepreneurs are working to make the dining industry more personalised. In the future I am sure that every dine-out experience will keep our blood glucose levels as predictable as a proper meal at home. Even today, though, we are already in a situation where we don't have to stay at home because we wish to avoid shaky sugars; eating out is becoming as manageable as eating at home. With more restaurants offering wider menus and displaying information about individual dishes, this trend is only going to grow. Interestingly, these changes are all helping to fuel a greater awareness about what we put into our bodies and what a difference eating balanced and nutritious meals can make *whether or not* you have diabetes.

From my experience, I think the dining industry is doing a superb job catering for the needs of people with special dietary requirements. We live in an age of so many different ways of eating. Most menus have an array of options, such as vegan, vegetarian, gluten free, nut free, dairy free and so on.

I don't see myself as someone with special dietary requirements and I don't think people with diabetes should have their own options on menus. At the end of the day, we should all be eating healthy food in its unrefined, natural form. If we just eat real food in its natural form, it makes insulin dosing significantly easier and safer.

Hidden oils, chemicals, sugars and so on shouldn't just be worrisome for people with diabetes. *Everyone* should be avoiding those things. If we all ate more plants and less processed food, we'd be thriving.

Drew Harrisberg, physiologist, model and singer-songwriter, Australia

5

ACTIVITIES

Yes, you can!

People ask me if I've ever thought I can't do something because of diabetes. I'd say the opposite is true. Diabetes has pushed me to do things I probably wouldn't have ever done. For example, I was a contestant on Australian Ninja Warrior and was the first person with Type 1 diabetes to ever hit the buzzer (atop a tough invisible-ladder challenge)! I missed out on a grand final spot by one place. I wanted to prove to myself and the world that diabetes isn't the only obstacle I can conquer.

Drew Harrisberg, physiologist, model and singer-songwriter, Australia

YES, YOU CAN DO IT!

From Kornelia's love of surfing to Josu's passion for climbing to Eoin's thing for weightlifting to Miguel's attraction to racing and Jonny's desire to keep dancing, I have heard it all. I will be brave enough now to state it as a fact: you can still exercise and enjoy sports very much if you have Type 1 diabetes. This is, as I have learned, a pretty good thing. Why? Well, while diabetes can occasionally be frustrating and inconvenient, it is often the very catalyst that drives you on to do more. Whatever activity it is that you love, a diagnosis never prevents you from pursuing an ambitious exercise routine.

If you are reading this and thinking 'Not me – I hate exercise', let me share a little of my own experience of what it feels like to have high blood sugar. This is something I am often asked about, since ordinary people simply don't experience it. As we've already seen in this book, when you have Type 1, your blood sugar will rise if the amount of carbs you consume is more than the equivalent amount of insulin you have in your body. It doesn't happen often, but when it does, I feel very odd. It is rather like having a little fluffy monster appear inside me. This creature gorges itself on my energy, ambition and curiosity, leaving me feeling a bit tired, disorganised and thirsty (little bastard!). I hate to even admit this to myself, but this is when I feel heavy and beaten. So, what am I compelled to do when this monster is taking over? Run! No, really. All I want to do is run. After a great deal of trial and error, I discovered the very best way to erase this internal terrorist is to perform physical activities. Running into the outside world is my personal tool to beat that fluffy monster. Injections are effective, but they don't solve the problem immediately.

Running does, or at least fairly rapidly. I really don't care if it is sunny, windy, wet or even snowing – I just want to feel the wind in my hair and run until I feel free again. And… magic! After a couple of kilometres and some kick-ass tunes (#AC/DC), I feel not only free of the restraining feeling but also proud and fulfilled. I have beaten the blood glucose monster down. The feeling of getting your blood glucose back on track is a moment of empowerment for every diabetic I've ever spoken to. It makes me feel like Superwoman or Lara Croft, ready to take on my next mission as if nothing has happened. My exercise has resolved my immediate problem of the blood-sugar high and I am back to normal. Plus, of course, I'm a little closer to my fitness goals!

> Being active during the week has a great impact on my diabetes management. It helps my blood sugar to be more stable and I don't need to take as much insulin for the food I am eating. Also, it is easier for me to eat carbs!
>
> I like to run as it helps me clear my mind, and I like to do strength workouts to build more muscle and to feel strong again. I always have some glucose tablets with me to be safe and to be able to continue my workout.
>
> *Sara Mobäck, influencer, Sweden*

It is quite possible that you will not embrace my technique for blasting away that blood-sugar high and will find your own coping mechanisms. That's fine. I would, however, urge anyone to consider exercise as an important part of their diabetes management routine, as well as their general wellbeing. Exercise has many advantages over and above pure fitness. It can help you lower your blood pressure and bad cholesterol, it lifts your mood, it beats stress and it improves your sleep patterns. Exercise is also handy in bringing down post-meal sugar spikes. Perhaps most importantly of all, it increases insulin sensitivity. You may be able to adjust your insulin levels because you've moved to a position of needing less insulin for a similar amount of carbohydrate than previously. It doesn't take long to have an effect either. You should start to notice a difference after just one or two days of exercise.

Yes, you can!

My favourite activity is going to the gym to work out, which I do every day with a mixture of weights, cardio and HIIT exercises (high-intensity interval training). I have always enjoyed this form of exercising, as I love to stay fit and have my body a certain shape. I've been doing it for about eight years now and still enjoy it just as much. I love to get in there and push my body. It has always been a great way for me to reduce stress, clear my head and keep healthy.

Diabetes plays a huge part in my sports and activity routines. It is essential for me and other diabetics to stay fit and healthy while living with this condition. Having diabetes gives you more of an incentive to look after your health and stay active. It's easy for people to take their health for granted, and I feel that if you're diagnosed with diabetes you become more aware of how fragile your health can be, and therefore more appreciate of being active. If you're not active, your diabetes is going to be a lot more difficult to manage. When we exercise and have a steady routine, we become more sensitive to insulin and therefore require smaller insulin doses. Exercising will also help to suppress food cravings. When we have less food cravings, we won't automatically reach for 'bad' foods. We are more conscious of what we're putting into our bodies and more likely to choose healthier options.

Eoin Costelloe, personal trainer and model, Ireland

FIND AN ACTIVITY YOU LOVE

I definitely have my parents to thank for doing their research and getting this all figured out. They pushed me to undertake numerous physical activities from day one. In fact, when I was very small, it often felt like they came up with a new sporting alternative *every time* they popped their head around my door. Thanks to their creativity, I've experienced an entire range of hobbies from swimming and gymnastics to sprint running and roller skating. They were never afraid to expose me to any of it. Their goal was clearly to impress upon me that diabetes is not an obstacle to any kind of sports activities. In fact, they positively discouraged me from compensating for my high blood sugar with an extra dose of insulin. 'Sports are the key to steady health and happiness' was something they said to me many times.

Activities

The fact that my parents always believed that I could do anything meant I never doubted it either. Yes, sometimes I had lows – occasionally even very bad lows – and sometimes I had highs. But it was all so natural that I never ever considered that I should stop digging for new experiences and learn new skills.

There were a few years when I didn't appreciate my parents' efforts. This happens to all children growing up, when they start to reach for independence of thought and action. For a while, I became lazy and disinterested and thought it was much more engaging to play computer games. My parents didn't let me off the hook, though, and persisted with their list of activities to try. And they did get through. They made me fall in love with exercise of any kind and helped me see that it makes it easier to keep my blood sugars on track. Even today, I keep a strict routine of training every day, even though I don't pursue sports professionally. I run first thing and follow it with a cold shower, which gives me a great mental charge. Running is my number one technique for keeping my blood sugar under control. My morning run always makes a huge difference to my daily wellbeing and makes me feel able to achieve any goal I set myself. Nothing, not even a bad blood glucose level, can get in my way.

Like many people who are diagnosed with Type 1, the day-to-day management of diabetes became a huge part of my life, very quickly. I wanted to play basketball at a high level, and my doctors told me that as long as I took care of my diabetes, I would be able to chase whatever dreams I had for my life.

I try to exercise three to five times a week and my regular activities are basketball, weightlifting, golf and running. I do them because I enjoy them, and they keep me in good shape. Diabetes is always present, so it is a big part of my routine and I plan ahead for any activities I am doing. It's demanding, but it is getting easier thanks to technology. I used to have to test my blood glucose before basketball games in college and then again at half-time. This was before continuous glucose monitoring devices were widely used.

Rob Howe, entrepreneur and founder, USA

Yes, you can!

If you had met me as a child, you might never have guessed that I had Type 1. I used to eat a lot of sugar, because it was the only thing that could keep my blood glucose up as I was such an active, restless kid. From ice creams to caramel chocolate bars, I had them all and stayed extremely thin too, all thanks to constant movement. Why all the sugar? Well, our muscles consume more glucose when we are active, so the chances of a hypo are higher.

When I had my birthday parties, we always made sure we were going somewhere like an indoor playground, where everyone would be constantly in motion. I did this right up until I was around 12 and began to crave more sophisticated pursuits. This way I could always have all the desserts in the world and the sweetest cake *and* enjoy my birthday just as any child should, *without an extra insulin shot.*

My constant jumping and running made my muscles work and enabled me to satisfy my sweet tooth, but they did give my mum a few headaches. When non-diabetics exercise, their bodies automatically reduce the amount of insulin they produce. This doesn't happen for people with Type 1, who don't produce insulin at all. We therefore need to take charge of adjusting our own levels, keep a watchful eye on our blood glucose levels and be aware of hypos during activities. But, hey, there is an upside. During and before physical activities is a great time to allow ourselves some foodie delights that we wouldn't otherwise have at other times.

One of the main reasons why biking is one of my favourite activities is because of my diabetes. I love being active and training, but it can be hard to find opportunities to measure my blood glucose while I'm working out. But, during long-distance biking, it is easier for me to keep a good blood glucose level and at the same time push myself. I also enjoy gym activities, such as body pump, spinning classes, HIIT training and weightlifting. I'm studying to be a PE teacher, so I practise lots of sports in school as well: volleyball, dance, tennis, skiing, swimming and so on. A couple of days a month I may have to cancel a gym class if I see that my blood glucose is sinking very fast. But most of the time I try to plan my activity so that my blood glucose is a bit higher than usual just before I start.

Elin Sandström, health and PE student and influencer, Sweden

DIFFERENT EXERCISES, DIFFERENT EFFECTS

Believe it or not, whichever sport I pursued, be it running, golf or dance, if I ever entered a competition, I never had to eat beforehand. This was because my stress levels were up in the skies, and they took my sugar there with them too. After some time as a diabetic, you'll realise that stress is a factor to watch out for in every part of your life, and it can definitely kick in during team and competitive activities in particular. There is no shame in succumbing to some pre-match nerves. Most people do, with or without Type 1. Stress releases a hormone that can impact our blood glucose, making it harder to keep on top of. I experienced the same thing during school exams and driving lessons. My blood glucose levels would always be up in the skies by the time I finished an assessment. I always think I should inject beforehand, but I never do as I figure it is better to finish with a lifted blood glucose than to interrupt the assessment time treating a low.

When doing Latin American dancing, my fellow dancers and I used to perform in front of huge audiences, and here my biggest childhood stress factor came into play: stage fright (I am not a natural performer). The Latin dance steps were incredibly fast moving and intense, but were interspersed with short periods of less movement as the coach 'walked' us through the routines. Added to this was the stress of trying to please the very strict coach. I was always careful to check my blood glucose levels right before I went on stage, though. I didn't want to end up in an emergency situation where I'd need to stop mid-set.[5]

Blood glucose planning can very much depend on the type of sport you pursue. It is crucial to plan beforehand for the activity you are embarking on because different types of exercise will have different impacts on your blood sugar levels. You might do anaerobic exercise, which involves high-intensity activity over a short period – for example, weightlifting, skipping, biking or HIIT. Alternatively, there is aerobic (cardio) exercise, which is lower in intensity but carried out over a longer period; examples include spinning, long-distance running and dancing. In my own case, when I did

---

5 *After 20 years with Type 1, I still haven't had my magic moment related to stress to enable me to completely overcome or ignore it. It is one of those things that happens occasionally that is totally beyond our control. We shouldn't beat ourselves up about it if and when it happens. If you have any suggestions on how to get on with it, or your personal tips and tricks, I would be happy to hear your stories via Instagram (@kristinaloskarjova).*

Yes, you can!

dancing four times a week over a period of five years, figuring out my blood glucose routine was easy. I asked the coach what kind of training we would do before the lesson and compensated accordingly. Something I realised very quickly was that my dance coach was not really concerned about my diabetes. She certainly wasn't willing to make any allowances for it, but she made sure she understood my condition and cooperated whenever I asked for a certain training type to make my blood glucose predictable. What bothered her most was to make sure that my classmates and I were always present at the lessons, followed her routines carefully and never questioned her! I certainly got the same treatment and criticism of my poor performance as everyone else in the group.

Since that time, I've mostly been involved in cardio workouts and know how they work on my body. To learn more about the relationships between exercise type and blood glucose levels, you could look up some of the participants in this book on social media, such as Eoin, Evan or Lauren (you can find their Instagram handles at the end of this book). I am sure they would be happy to help you with their professional advice. Also, make sure to speak to your healthcare team and your coaches. With this support, you will easily build up a routine that consists of the exercise types you enjoy.

One thing is for sure: you can always choose an activity you love and enjoy. In the process, you will figure out your body's reaction and adjust your treatment plan accordingly. I promise that, in the end, it will all become a natural, effort-free routine.

> With diabetes you can do anything really. You can. It's more of a mindset thing than an actual physical thing because, if you look after yourself and don't let too much into your brain about the limitations that you think that you've got ahead of you, you'll be fine.
>
> I've obviously had my trials and tribulations with my job. Sometimes I have periods of quiet and sometimes I jump into a show where I'm doing eight performances a week, dancing and all the rest of it. So, yeah, sometimes it's quite hard to manage my levels. Then there is food to be taken into account, which is affected by exercise and vice versa. I guess it's just a trial-and-error thing, but it's never really stopped me

from doing anything. I've never had to take time out or give up on anything. I refuse to let it happen like that. Maybe that's just me being stubborn.

Jonny Labey, actor, UK

Another sport I tried at the same time as dancing was golf. I admit, I knew very little about golf when my brother first came home and announced that he'd been golfing with his mates. I was curious enough to give it a try, though.

Golf is a very physical sport, requiring a great deal of stamina. When playing 18 holes, it's likely that you will walk for four or five hours straight, often over very uneven terrain. Initially, my blood glucose levels sank very low indeed and finding a way to even them out was tough. I persisted, though. I loved the sport, possibly for much the same reason I enjoy running so much: it is a brilliant way to get loads of fresh air, while enjoying nature and some fantastic scenery. It wasn't long before I became completely addicted to golf and played five times a week. It took me a couple of years to master taking care of my blood glucose levels while out on the course, but I manged it eventually. I need to be very organised and find the right routine, but it is well worth it.

I credit golf with teaching me my most important lesson about Type 1: diabetes is my best friend, sweetest partner and strictest teacher. It's always by my side, making me happy when I'm in a good mood and delivering a tough lesson when I make a mistake. It is also very loyal, so it is better to make sure to love and understand the condition, and not fight against it. Please forgive my moment of reflection: that's what you get for many, many hours wandering the greens!

The key for any Type 1, doing whatever type of exercise they prefer, is to test before, after and during exercise. There are plenty of studies to show that there are huge variations in how people react and respond to relatively similar activities. This makes guidelines useful, but certainly not the last word.

Yes, you can!

I wear a Dexcom glucose monitoring system, which helps a ton. It checks my blood sugar 24 hours a day, providing results on my phone and Apple watch. My goal is to have my blood sugar over 7.8 mmol/L (140 mg/dL) before driving, and I have never had a problem with it. The adrenaline raises my blood sugar on race days, so I have to have an extra dose of insulin most times, but it is not a big deal.

Miguel Paludo, champion racing driver, Brazil

DRIVING

I would like to highlight that, yes, we can drive a car and own a driving licence with diabetes. Indeed, I believe our car racing champion Miguel is a testament to this. Understandably, we do need to present a couple of extra doctors' notes when we apply for our licence and every country around the world has its own rules and regulations around that. But it's well worth putting in the effort. I love driving a car. In Hungary, the legal age for driving alone on the road is 18, but you can start driving lessons from the age of 17. I was so passionate about getting my licence that I started driving from the moment I was legally able to and was thrilled to see my driving licence arrive in the post on the actual day of my 18th birthday.

The impact of driving on blood glucose management is something else that everyone has to figure out for themselves. I haven't observed any unusual blood glucose behaviour while driving, except for when I drive on the highway or motorway, when my blood glucose usually skyrockets. I would suggest that this is due to the adrenaline that Miguel mentioned above. There is not much we can do about it, except for taking a break every hour or so by pulling over into a rest area along the highway to have a walking break. But again, these adrenaline spikes may simply be my own nervous reactions and your response might be different.

The only thing that we must not do is to start driving with (or into!) a hypo. Certainly, though, if you have ever dreamed about or looked forward to driving a car, diabetes is definitely not the reason to give up on this ambition.

(A side-note fun fact: just after I started taking driving lessons, my instructor's girlfriend was diagnosed with Type 1. You can imagine what the main topic of our discussions was during lessons and who received the most support!)

FIND THE MAGIC

How soon can you exercise after eating or work out before your meal? Timings are key. I discovered the joys of morning runs two years ago. For a long time, it felt challenging to slot time for sports into my daily university or work schedule. I rarely succeeded because I always seemed to choose a time when my blood glucose levels went off track during exercise, or the perfect time for measuring my blood glucose simply wasn't available. Then, I decided to experiment with doing sports early in the morning, before breakfast. And there was that magic I talked about earlier. It worked just perfectly and continues to do so today. It is the solution that feels truly natural. So natural, in fact, that I forget I have diabetes. This is when I know I have found my way.

I can't guarantee that a morning run will work for everyone. Some individuals find that their blood sugar spikes if they do sports at that time of the day. This could be down to the different insulin types used, the lifestyles we lead or simply our bodies' natural reactions to early morning activity. Our options are always greatly influenced by our own, personal readings. When, how and what sports we do is something we all need to figure out for ourselves by trial and error. However, diabetes is definitely never an excuse to miss out on the joy of activities!

Before you start making any drastic changes to your exercise routine, speak to your medical team to discuss insulin dosing and food compensation. Exercise affects everyone differently. Then, find out what works for you and stick with it.

My first big climb was Mont Blanc. I was 16 years old, but I didn't know then that I was diabetic. I was diagnosed when I was 23 years old. Since then, I have climbed Everest, which had been my dream since I was 8 years old, as well as many other peaks that no diabetic had ever attempted before. The fact that I was the first meant I had no references. Before each trip, I try to simulate the different situations that I am going to face in these other environments. This way, when I do it in a real situation, my diabetes is not a problem for me or my colleagues.

My advice to anyone who doesn't believe they can succeed, or do x, y or z because they have diabetes, is to simply listen

Yes, you can!

> to the people who know more than them. Speak to your endocrine doctors or talk to other diabetic patients who have already done the stuff you are being told you can't do. Then do it.
>
> *Josu Feijoo, mountaineer and astronaut, Basque Country*

I will leave you with one final thought on activities. A mentor once told me, 'Once you conquer yourself, you can conquer the whole world.' And it stuck with me. If you have Type 1 diabetes, I know you are conquering yourself every single day. However, have no doubts. The whole world is waiting for you. Be brave! Be active! And enjoy the magic that the world of activities has to offer.

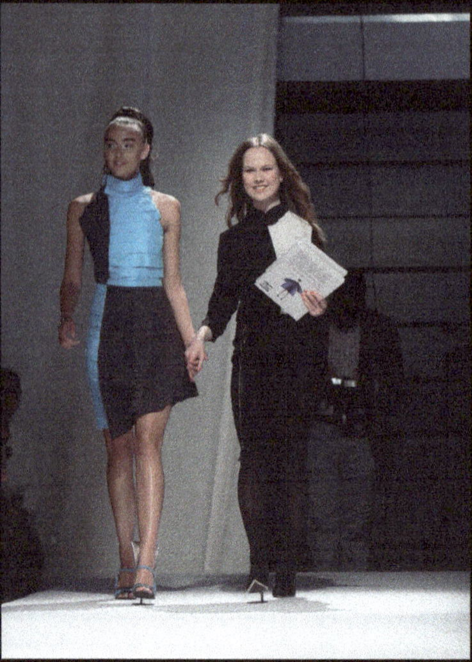

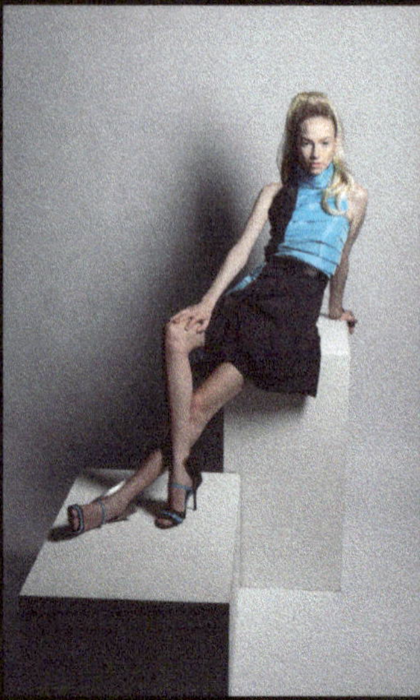

Yes, you can!

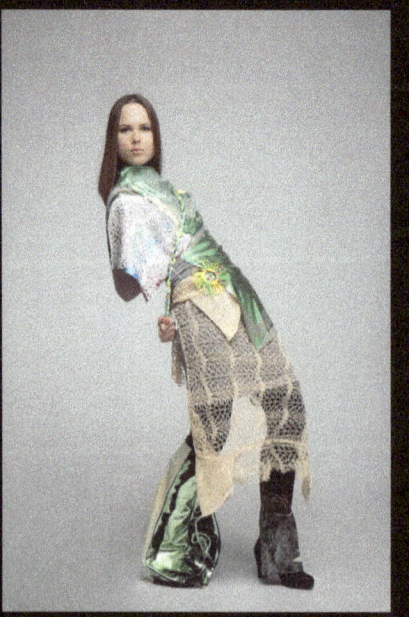

Winning the fashion competition at Regent's University (2016)

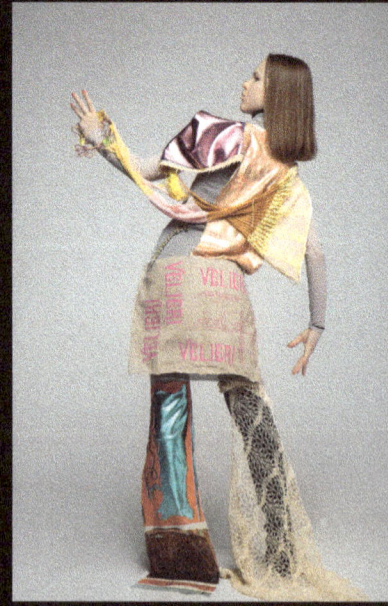

Modelling for a project at Central Saint Martins
(designs by Gina Grünwald @ginagrnw) (2019)

Kristina Loskarjova

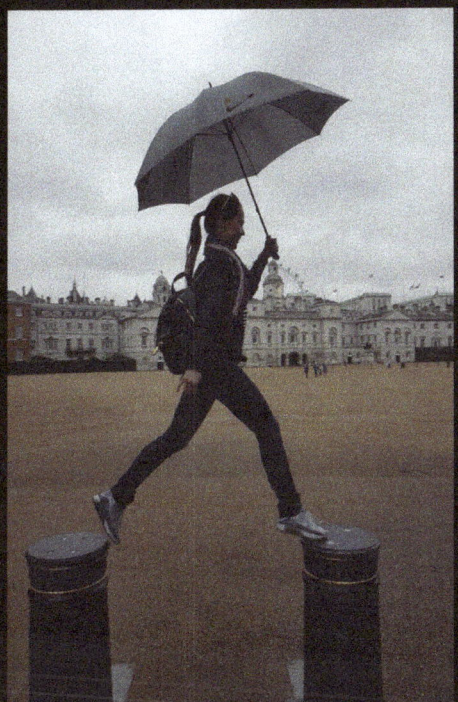
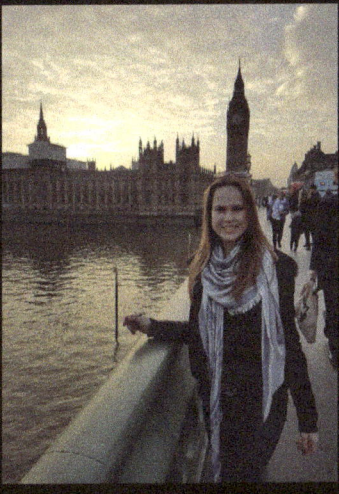

First time in London (2016)

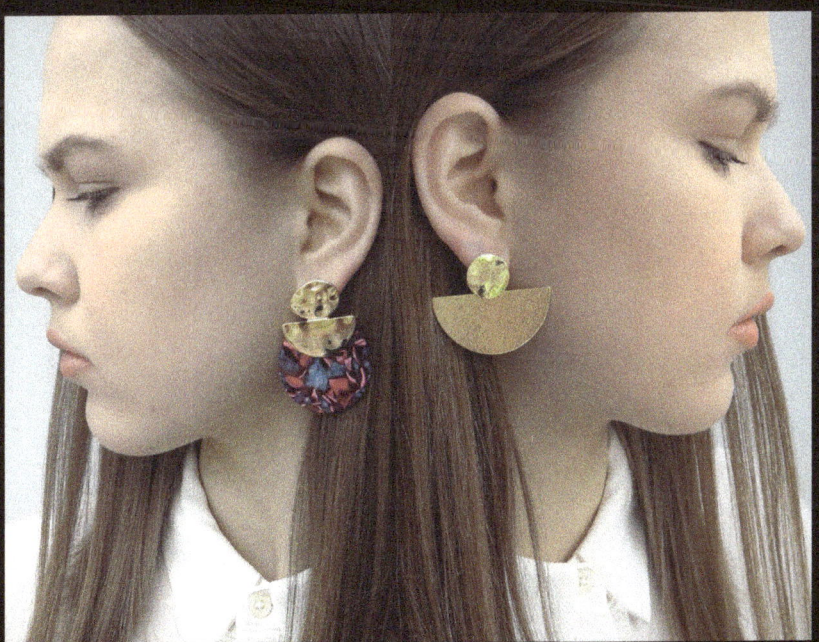

A marketing campaign for my Connfience earring store (2018)

Yes, you can!

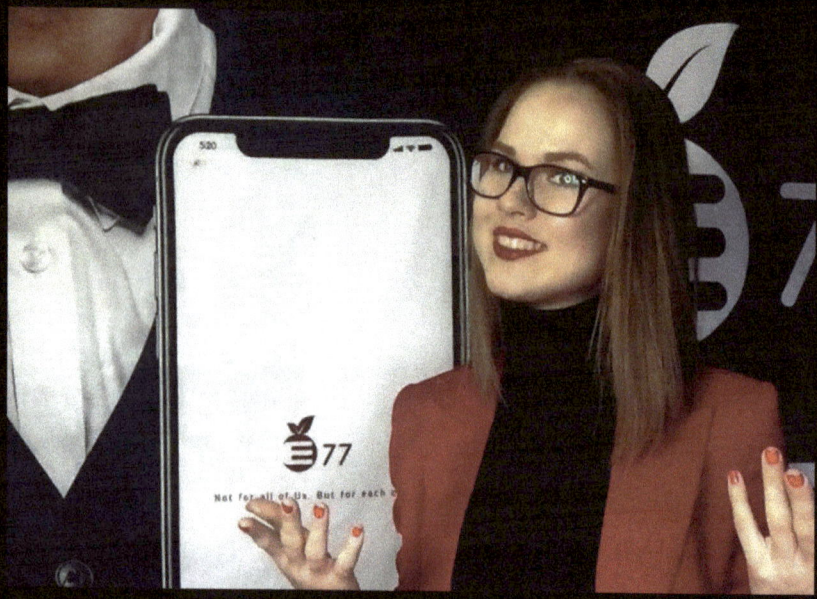

Presenting for my current venture E77 (www.e77.io)

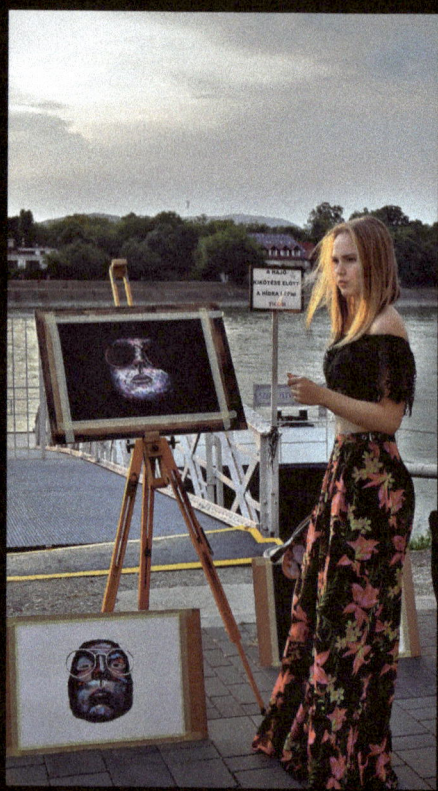

Drawings (2019)

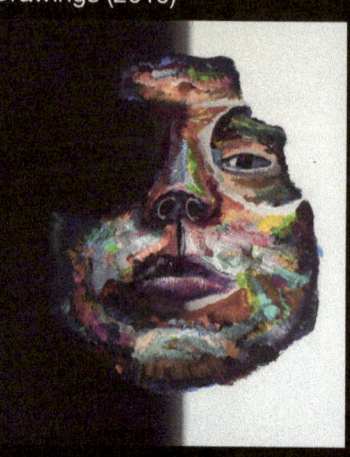

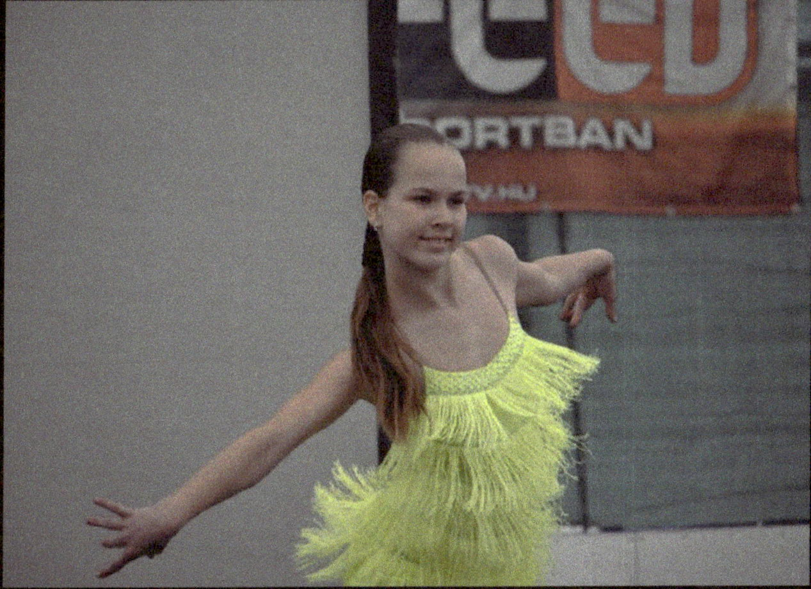

Performing on stage when I was doing Latin-American dance (2011)

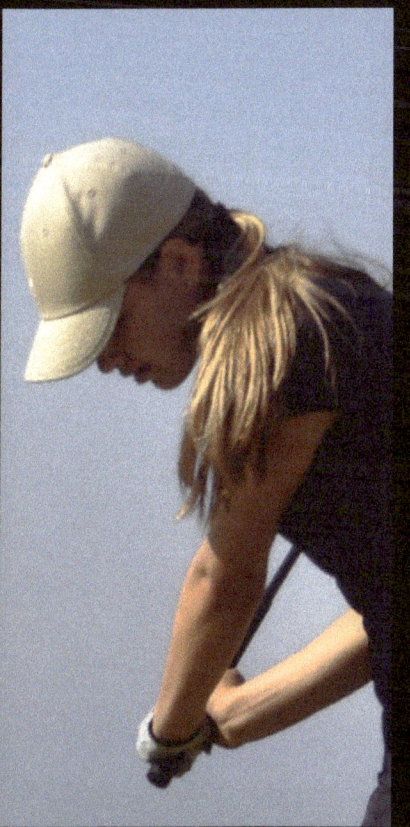

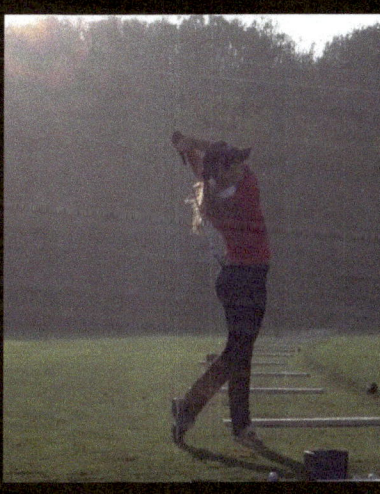

Playing golf (2013)

Yes, you can!

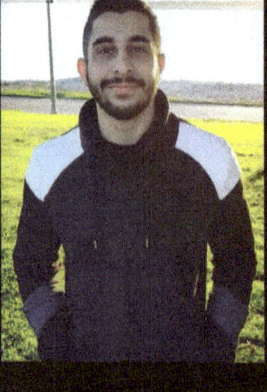

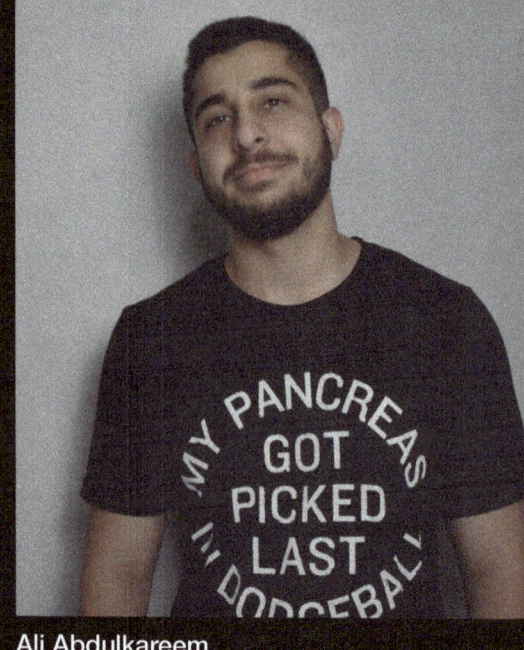

Ali Abdulkareem,
Blogger and job coach, USA

David Mina,
Graphic Designer, USA

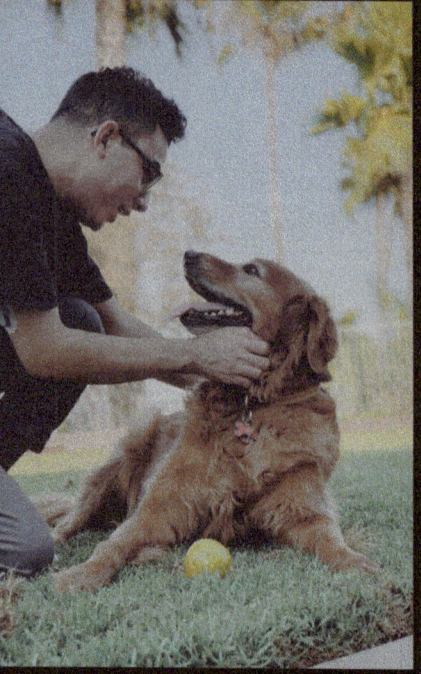

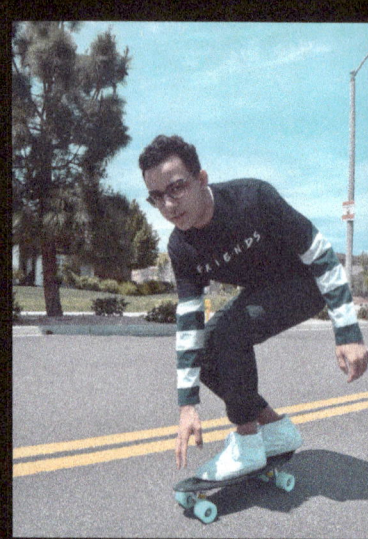

Ali, David, Drew and Eoin

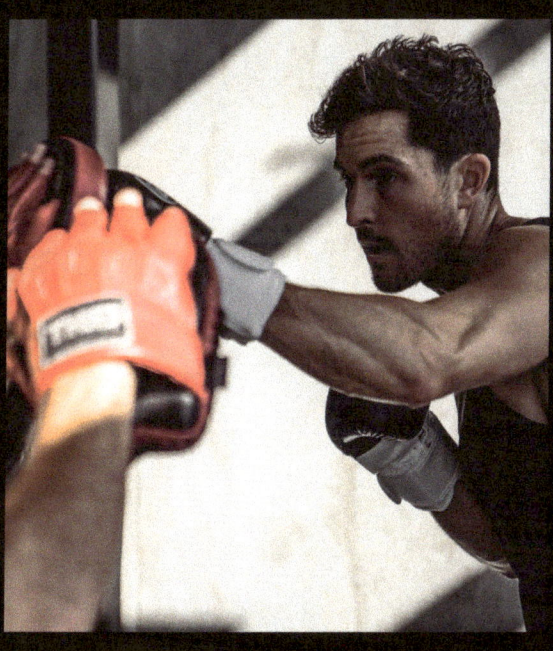
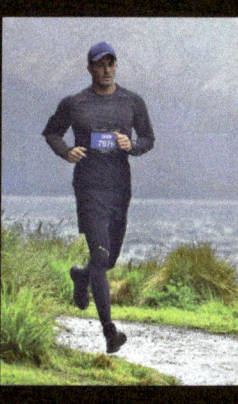

Drew Harrisberg,
Physiologist, Model And Singer-Songwriter, Australia

Eoin Costelloe,
Personal trainer and model, Ireland

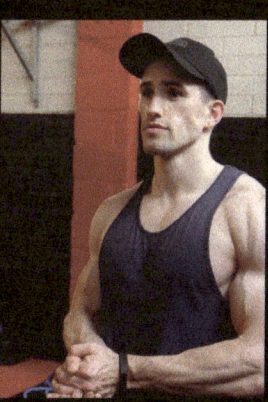
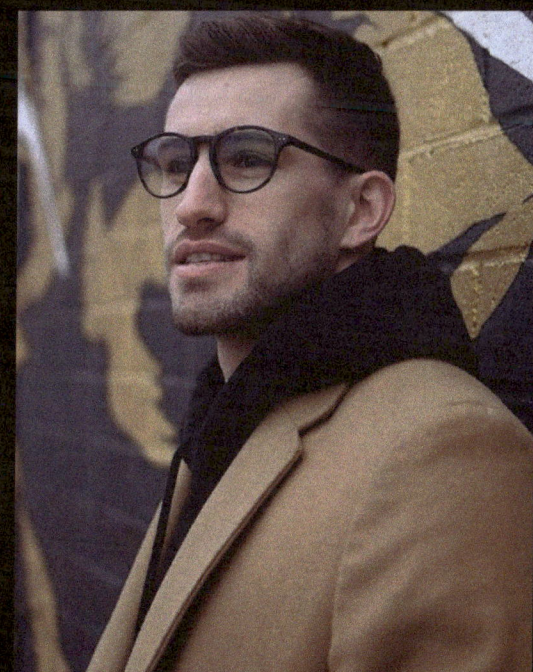

Yes, you can!

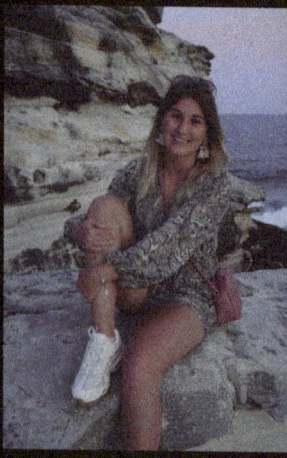

Elin Sandström,
Health and PE student and influencer,
Sweden

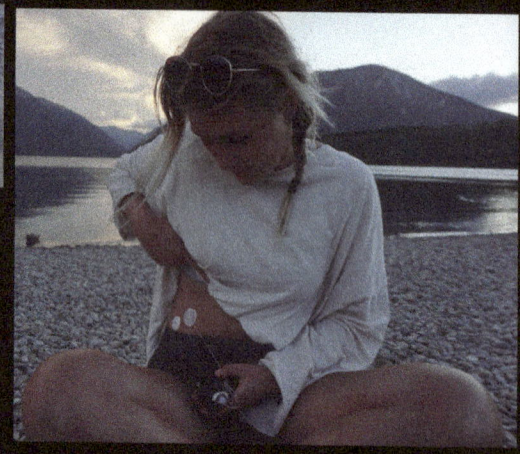

Evan Soroka,
Yoga therapist, USA

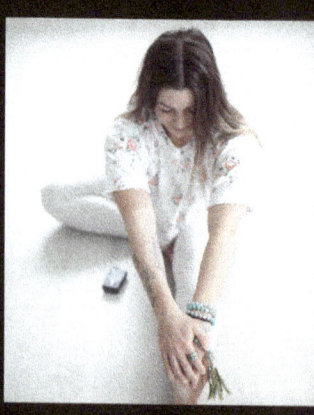

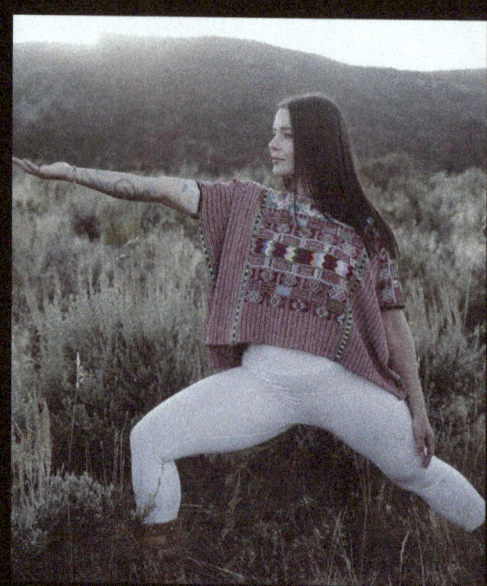

Elin, Evan, Jonny and Josu

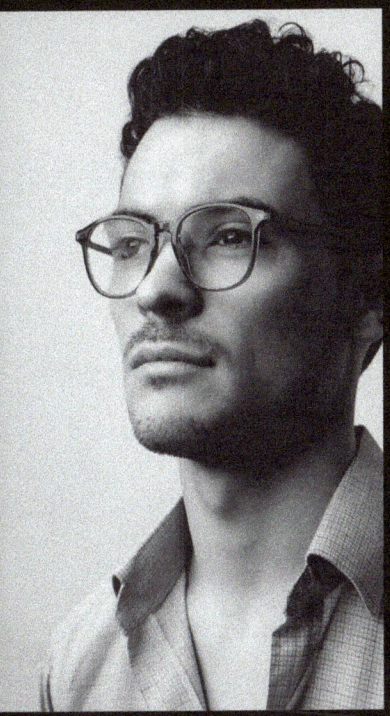

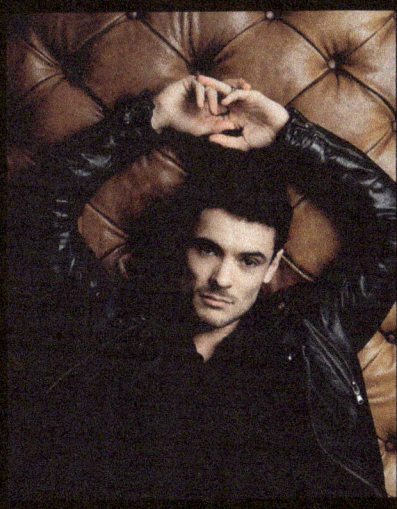

Jonny Labey,
Actor, UK

Josu Feijoo,
Mountaineer and astronaut, Basque Country

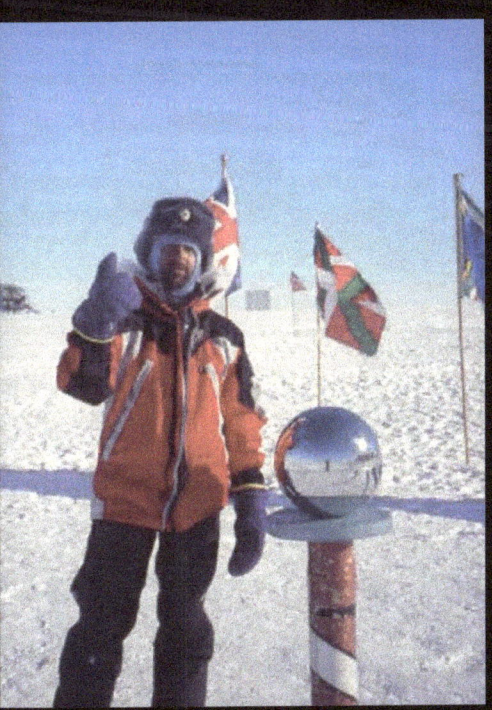

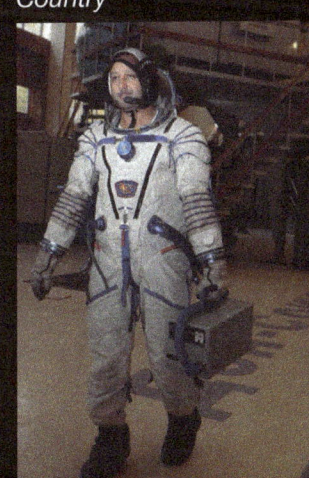

Kornelia Mango,
Singer and celebrity, Russia

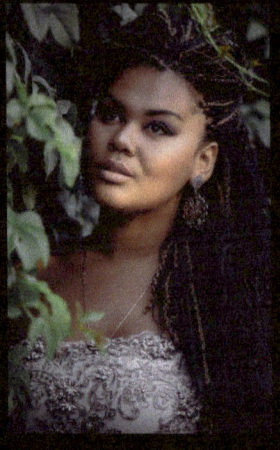

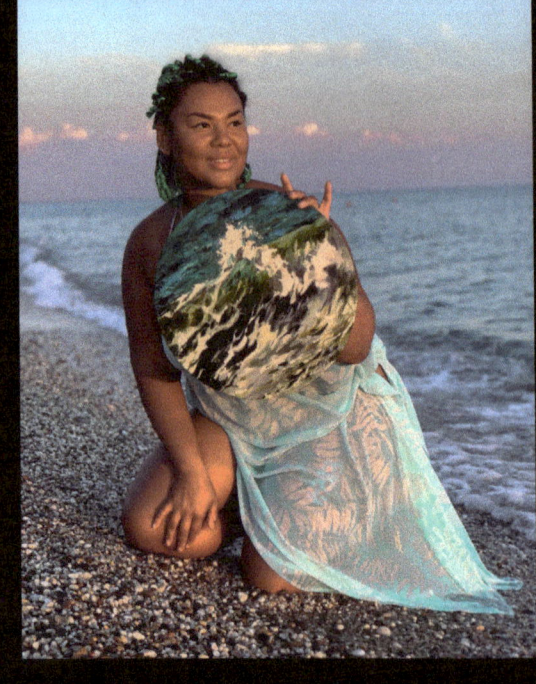

Lauren Bongiorno,
Diabetes health coach, USA

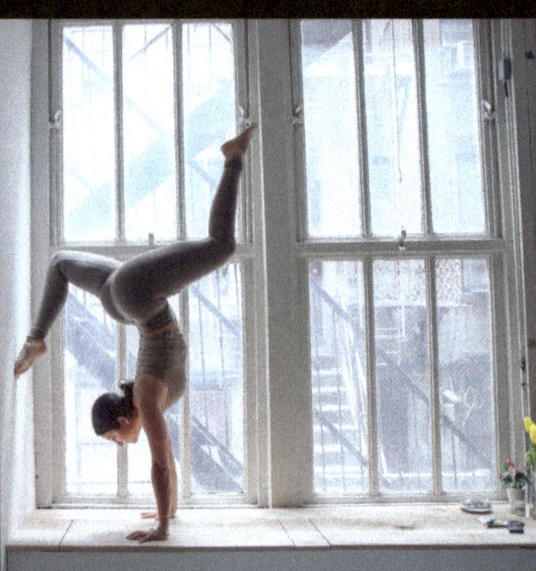

Kornelia, Lauren, Matt and Miguel

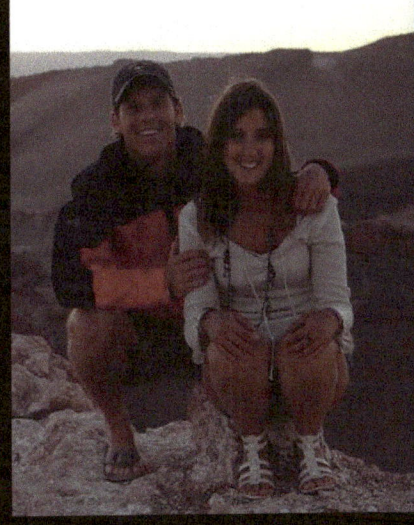

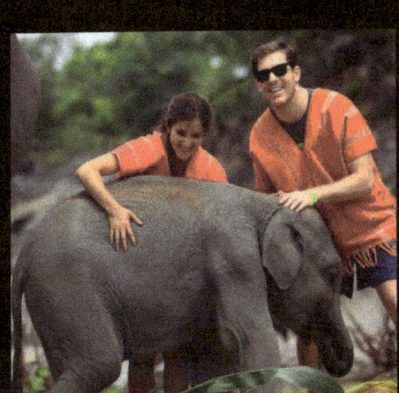

Matt Collins,
Robotic surgery business leader, USA

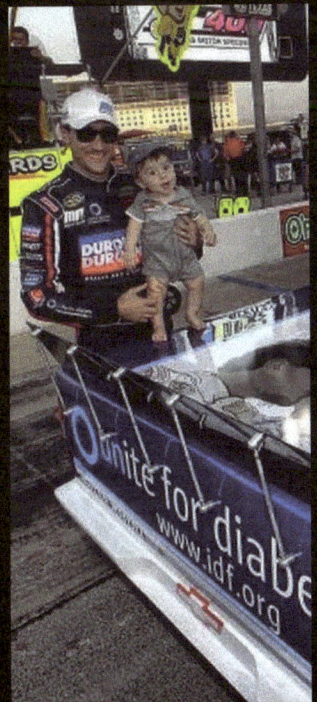

Miguel Paludo,
Champion racing driver, Brazil

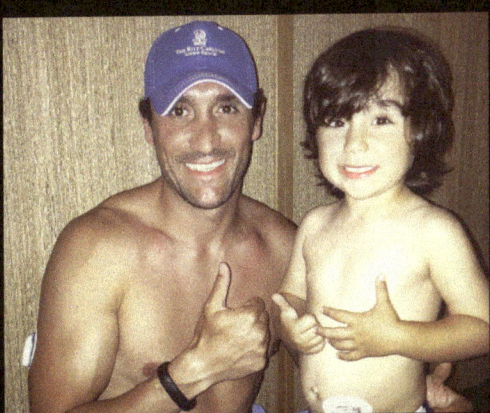

Yes, you can!

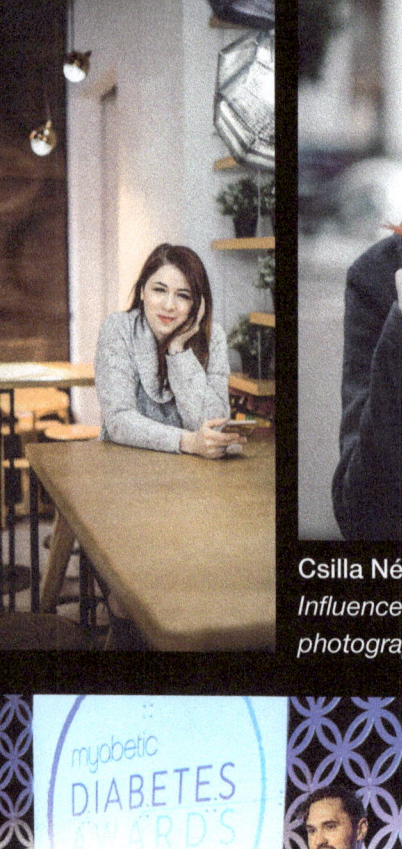

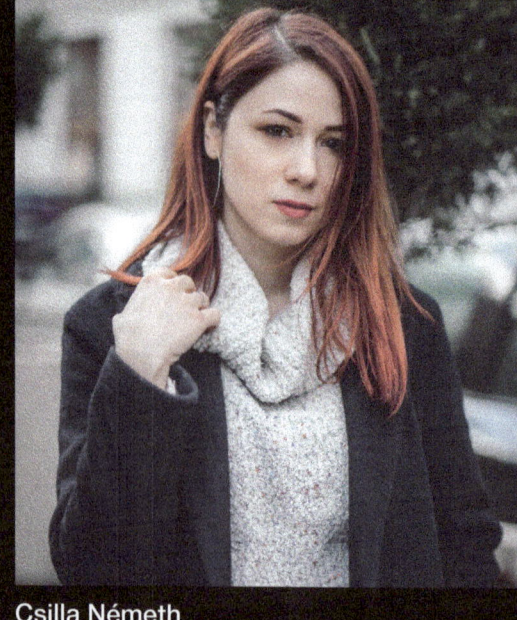

Csilla Németh,
Influencer, blogger and photographer, Hungary

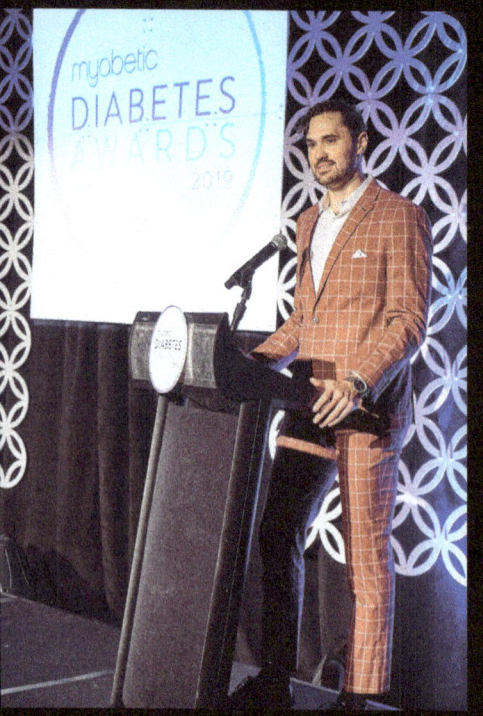

Rob Howe,
Entrepreneur and founder, USA

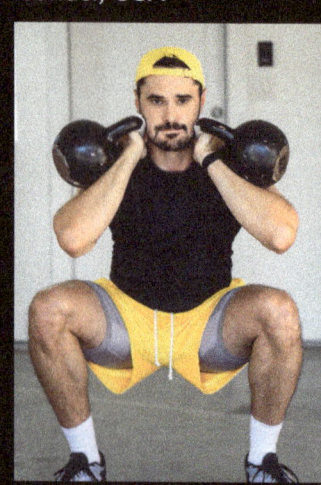

Csilla, Rob, Sara and Stephen

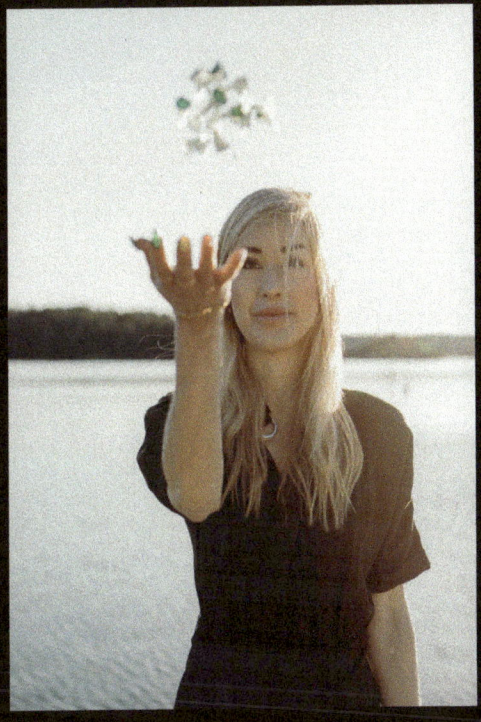

Sara Mobäck,
Influencer, Sweden

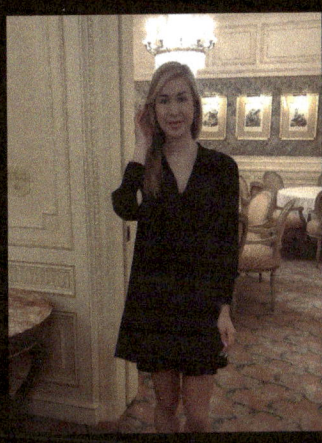

Stephen Dixon,
*Sky News
presenter, UK*

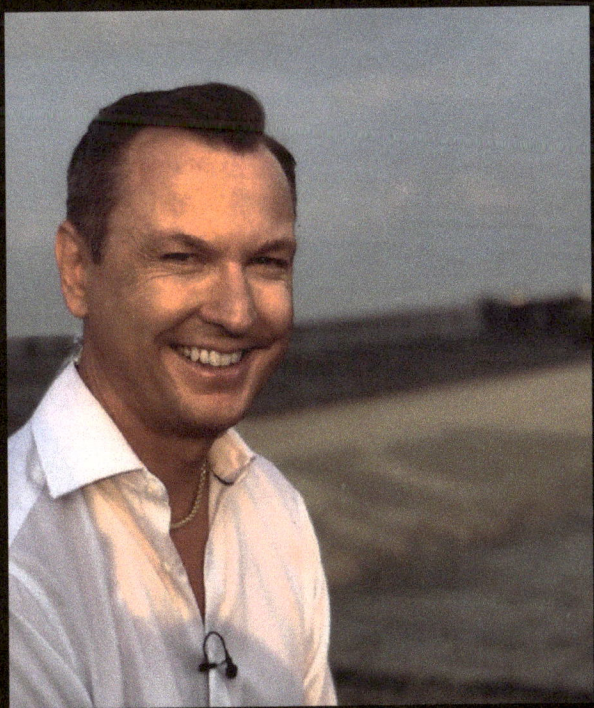

6
TRAVELLING

Yes, you can!

I had been really excited about a family vacation to the beautiful island of Honolulu, Hawaii. I've always been obsessed with anything that's related to the tropics or sandy beaches. The night before we went, I was really careful to pack everything. I had a separate backpack with all my diabetes supplies packed, except for my insulin, which needs to be in the fridge when it is not being used. My plan was to grab it in the morning and add it to the backpack just before I left for the airport with my family. You can guess what happened next. I completely forgot to pick it up.

The worst thing was, I only discovered my mistake when we reached the airport, which was a near two-hour journey from my house. The flight was about to board and there was no time to go home, or even to go to the nearest pharmacy. As anyone with Type 1 knows, we can't live without insulin. It's like being a fish out of water. Part of me was disappointed in myself for forgetting it. An even bigger part of me was in a complete panic. When I told my parents, I could see how shocked they were too. Luckily, my mom knew exactly what to do and swung into action. She called my endocrinologist and pharmacy and explained what was happening. They immediately put in an order for me at a pharmacy in Hawaii that was close to our destination. Fortunately, I wear a pump, and I had changed out my site the night before, filling a new reservoir. I had three days before it ran out, so I knew it would be OK during the five hours from California to Hawaii. If I hadn't been wearing a pump, I don't know what I would have done. It was all a bit stressful at the time, but it worked out OK.

David Mina, graphic designer, USA

TRAVELLING IS GREAT FOR *EVERYONE!*

I have always loved travelling, whether to cities around Hungary, to countries around Europe or even all the way to the vast and unforgiving Siberian territories of Russia. From when I was around 8 years old, my parents would confidently take me on a series of planes and then a couple of overnight train rides to get me to the villages where they came from. I used to call those villages 'the edge of civilisation'. The houses had no modern heating, there was no phone connection and no 3G or 4G data, and guess what… no Wi-Fi. Supplies of food, goods and medicine in the local store depended on the weather conditions. If there had been heavy rain and flooding, the transport (both trains and planes) supplying the items simply couldn't access the village. And, another fun fact, the toilets were all located *outside* the houses. They were pretty basic too. Certainly, there was no fancy flushing as the water supply was not designed that way.

These various hardships would be tough on any 21st-century child, but especially so for one with diabetes. When access to water and medicine is as important as breathing air, such conditions are particularly challenging. Yet, I spent some of the happiest moments of my childhood in those villages. The combination of fresh air, pure nature and the lack of tech truly energised me. My brother, cousins and I fished, swam and helped harvest our grandparents' crops. We even hunted! The purpose of most of the activities was to get food and maintain life, not for fun, but we loved it all. My blood glucose levels were never as good as when I spent time in Siberia. I barely noticed that in our free time we couldn't play computer games or browse social media. Card games, sports activities and creativity were all we had.

The experience led me to one conclusion: travelling is great for everyone, including Type 1s. To enjoy these truly fulfilling experiences, plan ahead and stock up on supplies so they last for a longer time than your actual trip. This will prepare you for any possible unexpected situation. That's really it. Diabetes certainly shouldn't curb your wanderlust in any way.

PLAN AND PREPARE

I like taking the odd risk and being spontaneous, but I never do this when it comes to packing. In fact, I always overpack but this is why, in 20 years of travelling, I've never run out of medical necessities. Overcautious? Maybe, but it makes sense to take extra care when preparing for travel as a Type 1, particularly when you know that you'll be absent for a certain period of time. We need to make sure we have enough insulin to cover the period we are away. It might be challenging to find insulin in a foreign country.

Most people's checkbox of essential travel items looks like this:
- Wallet
- Passport
- Phone

Yes, you can!

The equivalent checkbox for a diabetic (based on my experience) looks something like this:
- Insulin pens (or pump)
- Extra needles
- Extra insulin (to cover the time of the stay)
- Continuous glucose monitoring (CGM) device (sensor and transmitter)
- Glucose meter (in case the CGM fails to work) and strips for the meter
- Emergency hypo food (during travel, this is especially important)
- Wallet
- Passport
- Phone (and, if you wear a CGM, possibly a second phone, to make sure that even if one stops working for any reason, you always have a backup)

Write your own checklist according to the supplies you use and go through it before leaving for every trip. It might seem like a hassle, but it's definitely better than realising that you forgot something half way through your travels.

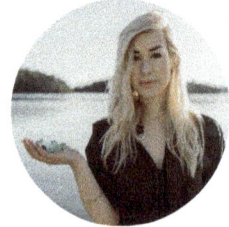

The funniest thing about a pump is security in airports. When I was wearing one, it always set off the alarms. Security always asked me to take the pump off and I had to explain why it was not a good idea to do so.

Sara Mobäck, influencer, Sweden

Researching your destination on the internet is always a lot of fun and builds up the anticipation. Check out the climate, the places you'd like to visit and what your accommodation looks like. Have one eye on how the location might affect your blood sugar, or your diabetes equipment, but you always need to do that when you go out at home anyway. Likewise, map out local pharmacies and other facilities in case of emergency, but again: nothing new. Same routine but *much more exciting* surroundings.

Checking out how much sun, or snow, to expect is a lot of fun. Remember too, though, a change in climate might result in differing blood glucose levels. And yes, you've guessed it, everybody reacts differently to every climate. I find a hot climate challenging for my daily routine. It immediately lowers my blood glucose, especially after a day in the sun, but my blood glucose might spike another day. In other words, it becomes very unpredictable and takes time to stabilise. Insulin is absorbed more quickly in hot weather, so you need to be more diligent than usual, monitoring your levels more often and adjusting your diet and insulin as required. Bear in mind that the quality of your insulin can deteriorate in hot weather. A cool bag can come in handy here.

When I am visiting mountains and colder climates, my blood glucose levels magically even out. Blood glucose management becomes significantly easier because insulin is absorbed more slowly in the cold. But this might also be because I enjoy mountains more than sunny beaches! You may be vulnerable to spikes here too, especially if you warm up later in the day by, say, nipping into an alpine cabin for a warm drink. Plus, your body uses up more energy when it tries to get or stay warm, so be aware of that.

The aim is to maintain a balance between enjoying your trip (which is what you are there to do) and remaining vigilant, just as you would at home. The main thing is to observe first and react accordingly. Oh, and don't get angry if things go a bit sideways in the first few days of travel. You're on holiday: relax!

When I was younger, I didn't really think about diabetes getting in the way of anything. So, aged 16, I said to my parents, 'I'm gonna go on an exchange and live in Brazil for year, in the middle of nowhere!' I did that. When I was in college, I was really into anthropology and primatology. I wanted to be a primatologist and part of that involved living in a secluded place in the jungle for months at a time. I realised pretty quickly that that was not going to be a reality with diabetes. There would be some things I couldn't do, even though there would be a lot of things I could do. I've adventured the world, though, and worked on archaeological digs all over Peru. I've travelled all over the jungle too. I've been to so many places and done a lot of stuff, like climbing huge mountains and testing my physical limits on my bike. Maybe I just like saying, 'I'm just gonna do it.'

Evan Soroka, yoga therapist, USA

Yes, you can!

ENJOYING YOUR TRIP IS THE PRIORITY

One of the most extreme journeys I ever took was with a high-school classmate of mine when I was 14 years old. Her family had invited me to join them on their annual summer trip to the mountain Grossglockner in Austria. Somehow, during the planning phase, no one mentioned that this was the highest peak in Austria and, to my and my suitcase's surprise, the temperature ranged between −3 and 3 degrees Celsius, even though it was the height of August. And, of course, it was snowing. I had to buy some not-too-trendy, yet essential, clothes from the local shop. Luckily, I was too excited about exploring nature to have much time to worry about my outfits. I felt warm and that meant we could start our trip!

The pure excitement of experiencing snow in August (something you don't necessarily experience in Hungary, even in winter) was what truly heated me up. We hiked for an entire week, up and down the uneven footpaths. Each time we got down from the peak of a mountain, my classmate's dad would joke, 'Kristina, don't you want to check your blood sugar? It must have dropped down by about 600 metres.' Everything was fine in that department, though, and the environment was breathtakingly beautiful. I didn't even consider how tiring the trip was, although the experience made me realise I had muscles in places I didn't know existed! It was like spending seven solid days in the gym and, I won't lie, I enjoyed quite a few sweets as my blood glucose levels tended to be on the low side.

Hiking was not the only activity. We also took a train to the nearest Italian city and then cycled back to Austria. We completed 60 km in just two hours. (The family were regulars at spin classes back at home, so even with my sports background I had to cycle really fast to make sure I was not left behind.) Of course, the cycling route was not a flat, straight one – that would have been too easy! It was all crazy, up and down hills, although at least it was tarmacked. I was not a fan of bikes at the time and didn't cycle often, and the new set of muscles I discovered reminded me of the experience for many, many days after the ride.

The final, fun climax of our trip was white-water rafting. I admit, I was a little scared about this one, but not because of diabetes, just in terms of my general survival. This was doubly so after we were told that the current could take us away if we fell out of the boat or it turned over. And this was supposed to be fun…?!? I didn't know what to think, so I just threw myself into the experience. I ate quite a lot beforehand, to make sure my blood glucose didn't fall, because measuring it in the rocky river would have been the last thing I wanted to do. If I recall well, the water was 2–4 degrees Celsius too, so I also concentrated heavily on heating my body up.

Clearly, I survived (and enjoyed every minute). What this trip proved is that when embarking on 'extreme' trips or activities, it is never diabetes that makes me scared. And rightly so. It would never be the reason why I declined a cool experience either. In fact, the only thing that would ever get the better of me and stop me taking another deep-dive moment would be my frayed nerves. So far, though, they've never let me down.

I travel a lot. In my experience, airports are the toughest places to find good food. Availability and access to good-quality food that I can confidently consume is a big problem. It's the time I get most uncertain about the amount of carbs in the food. This leaves me having to guess the amount of insulin that I inject.

Matt Collins, robotic surgery business leader, USA

FOOD, GLORIOUS (AND DIFFERENT) FOOD

Travelling is a more challenging version of eating out – you never really know what to expect. This is not only related to the different types of food you encounter, but also to the habits of the country in general. Not knowing certain details can result in very unexpected moments, as you will see from a few of my travel experiences.

The first one I will share came on a family trip to Italy. Our first stop for the night was a small village not far from the Slovenian border. We were all very excited about exploring and, in particular, eating. Italian food is said to be very good in the country's small towns, partly because this is where all the traditions are well kept. We arrived around midday and checked into our hotel before heading to our first, very much anticipated and desired, Italian lunch. My blood sugar was high at the time, but I was determined to have my fill of tasty Italian carbs, so I injected my insulin before I left the hotel room. Now, as you know, insulin needs time to be absorbed. We all eagerly headed to the pizzeria that we'd eyed up earlier on, only to discover it was closed. So, as it turned out, was every single other restaurant in the streets around us. At lunchtime, the entire town went on a siesta. And lunchtime lasted from 12.30 until 3pm! I needed

Yes, you can!

food ASAP, but nothing was open – not one shop – and I did not have enough emergency food with me. We tried multiple places, but everything was shuttered. Absolutely no one was around. The entire village looked like a ghost town. Eventually, we found a lost sandwich hidden on the back seat of our car. It was one that my mum had prepared before we left home. It was not the time to be a picky eater! I ate the sandwich in time and the problem was solved. Well, with the exception of my poor family, who had to wait until 3pm to get some food inside them.

It should be said, this scenario is unlikely to happen today. This was ten years ago, in the days before you could pull out a phone and check on opening times.

Another good lesson I learned was thanks to a breakfast in an Austrian hotel. The starting point of my mistake was similar. I injected in the room rather than in the actual dining place. Our rooms were on the fifth floor and we decided it was a good idea to take the stairs in case, for some reason, we got stuck in the elevator. This seemed prudent, since I had already injected and now all I needed was to get close to the buffet. Unfortunately, after we entered the stairwell, the door slammed behind us with an ominous thud. It was only then we discovered that the stair doors of the hotel could only be opened from the outside, which meant we were stuck… whoops. Instead of getting stuck in the elevator, we'd got stuck in the stairs area with no emergency food on us and no service on our phones. Brilliant.

Fortunately, we all kept our wits about us. I was fairly sure there must be a door somewhere that would get us back into the building and there was. A couple of floors below, we breezed through the tradespeople's entrance, into the kitchen. From there, after being given some very surprised looks from the kitchen staff, we were invited to enjoy the breakfast buffet, where I managed to get my food on time.

I think the lesson in both cases here is: always have emergency food on you. Always.

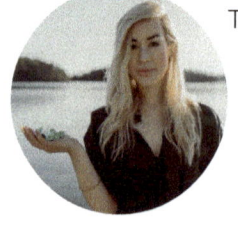

The biggest problem with any sort of restaurant, anywhere in the world, is the uncertainty. We can't always be sure of the carbohydrate count in the foods we order. I've got used to it, and most of the time I know roughly how many units of carbohydrates I eat, but there are times when I need to guess. Then there is the timing. As diabetics, we often find ourselves thinking, 'How much should I inject?' And, 'When is the food coming?' Timing for us is key and oftentimes, after submitting an order in a restaurant, we decide to inject our insulin dose to make sure that when the food arrives and we start to eat, the insulin is already working and our blood sugar doesn't spike from the food we eat. But, what if the service is 'relaxed'? Or, part of the order arrives, but it is the part without the carbs? Unfortunately, some restaurants are poorly organised and there can be cases where, when we order (for example) fish and potato, only the fish arrives. We always need to have emergency snacks in our bags for these kinds of moments.

Sara Mobäck, influencer, Sweden

When it comes to ordering food abroad, the menu choices will be different from what you are used to. And, as my final travel story will show, this can trip you up. On this occasion, I was in the Greek part of Cyprus. Interested in the local cuisine, I asked the waiters what meze was. Their response was that it was a traditional Middle Eastern meal. It sounded like exactly what I'd come for, so I confidently ordered a fish meze. When they brought the first course, a light veggie and sauce mix, I injected. Then came the second, slightly heavier course, which featured quite some carbs, and then the third, which was a selection of fish cuts. But there was more. The fourth course was pita breads, hummus and tahini, all in very generous portions. When the waiter collected my plate, I joked, 'Delicious! But I hope this is the last one!' The waiter looked confused before telling me that there were *eight more courses* on the way! *Excuse me?!* Meze is a 12-plate course, he quietly explained. (And yes, it is designed for just one person.) I couldn't believe it. Mind you, it was delicious. I haven't eaten such fresh food for a long time, but it definitely didn't fit in my stomach or my carb count! To cut a long story short (or rather, long dinner short), I had to share the food with my friends at the table. Luckily, their meals consisted of small portions, the ones that most people *usually* have for dinner. But isn't this the best part of eating food abroad with your mates? You can always share. Nevertheless, since

Yes, you can!

having this meal, I have always made a point of asking restaurants abroad what exactly they mean by 'traditional'.

> My greatest challenge is to travel around in any country other than those of Scandinavia. I have quite a healthy diet and, for me, breakfast is the most important meal of the day. I find it especially hard when you come to a hotel or hostel and they only serve white toast with jam and peanut butter. In the best case, they also have some yoghurt, but then it is often sweetened.
>
> The dining industry worldwide needs to be healthier overall – not just because of people who have special dietary requirements, but because obesity and other lifestyle diseases kill too many people! If the dining industry were healthier, it would be easier for everyone to be healthy, and easier for me, as a diabetic, to eat better food for my blood sugar.
>
> *Elin Sandström, health and PE student and influencer, Sweden*

The final point to make is not to be self-conscious. Just because you are in a strange place, it doesn't mean that no one has ever heard of Type 1. People all over the world have the condition. They may deal with it differently, but the sight of you with a pen is not going to blow anyone's mind, any more than it will for folks back home. Different people react differently and that will be the same on your travels regardless of where you go. Exercise the same strategies that you use at home when it comes to telling others and using your supplies.

> Instagram has been a great way of unifying our experiences of diabetes everywhere. It shows us that we are not the only ones out there, and I think that has been a massive transition for a lot of people all over the world. There are so many other people out there that are living just the same way.
>
> The response to diabetes varies from country to country. In South America and Europe, for example, people will ask me what stuff is. In America, people don't ask you at all. They might look at it, but they don't ask. In America, everyone's

so politically correct. They're like, 'Oh you shouldn't call yourself *a* diabetic, you should call yourself *a person* with diabetes.' I have no problem calling myself a diabetic, but that's how it is for me.

I'm proud to be a diabetic. I wear my pump visibly as a badge of honour. I'm not worried about the questions. I actually appreciate it when people ask questions.

Evan Soroka, yoga therapist, USA

7
CAREERS

Yes, you can!

My mum sent me through a copy of my schedule and diary from the year after I was diagnosed (aged 15). If anything, my life got busier. I was in about five shows at the time. I had just got into the Dance World Cup and had won a couple of trophies. So, apart from the adjustment period, which was a couple of weeks off school and getting used to it, I was back at work. I just needed to be reassured that it wasn't going to affect my feet, or my dance career, and then I pretty much just got straight back in role.

I went on to play a character on *EastEnders* called Paul Coker. After meeting with the producers, I suggested that they gave my character diabetes and they went with it. They enjoyed that idea and that also led to my involvement with Diabetes UK, which later led me to creating my own diabetes-focused YouTube channel called Know Your Type. This basically meant going around interviewing all sorts of different inspirational Type 1 diabetics from different walks of life. It succeeded in representing diabetes on a more human level, as opposed to a statistical level. That, in turn, led to my new involvement with the researching team of JDRF, the biggest global diabetic charity, which has been exciting. I've met some incredible people and I've learned some incredible things.

Jonny Labey, actor, UK

YOUR CAREER, YOUR CHOICE!

Careers are just like activities: you are in control of your choice. What you do fully depends on your aspirations. Type 1s with incredible careers include Damon Dash, the music mogul behind Roc-A-Fella Records, which helped to launch Jay-Z and Kanye West to fame; actress Halle Berry; Silicon Valley software CEO Steve Lucas; and *Vampire Chronicles* author Anne Rice – to name but a very few. Each one has reached the peak of their profession and is a brilliant role model for what any of us can achieve. You may, as many people in this book have done, make a career out of your condition. There are plenty of opportunities for yoga instructors, personal trainers and influencers, all of whom can help fellow Type 1s while doing important work to spread the word.

Diabetes should never get in the way of anything you want to do. When properly managed, it is part of you – part of your life – and that is it. What you choose to do with that life is entirely up to you. In fact, your diagnosis might even spur you on to achieve even *more* than you ever imagined. I certainly feel that way and many, many of the Type 1s I have spoken to have said as much.

When it comes to who we want to be, how we wish to earn our money and how we want to live our life, the same principles largely apply to everyone, regardless of whether or not they have Type 1. I also feel that our blood glucose levels are best when we are fully engaged in whatever we like to do. This might sound like a very basic observation, but it shone through when I spoke to the inspiring individuals who contributed to this book (and whenever I speak to other Type 1s). Life is easier for us all when we earn our living doing something we enjoy. The trick is to adjust the condition to your lifestyle and never the other way around.

If you know what you really want to achieve in life, go for it and you will always be able to find a way to manage your diabetes around your goal. This might be by yourself or with your healthcare team, or even with the help of other diabetics in the same field as your chosen career path. We can always adjust our insulin and change our treatment. If you think about yourself as a car for a moment (remember that wonderful manual car from the beginning of this book?), you can take action to tune up your imperfect car engine in a way that makes it possible and convenient for you to drive to your desired destinations. This is exactly what everyone has to do, Type 1 or otherwise. No one can drive a car that doesn't fit their skill set or size; they adjust the seating, sort out the mirrors and maybe personalise it by upgrading the vehicle with some innovative devices. All of this goes towards having the car in perfect condition for the road you decide to drive on. Diabetes is exactly the same. We don't have to choose the road according to the car; we can and should choose the road and drive the journey of our lives. Thanks to the times we live in, we can always adjust our blood glucose treatment to our needs and proceed happily to our chosen destinations.

Yes, you can!

> I try to manage my work in the same way as I manage my diabetes: by giving my best effort and being proactive.
>
> *Rob Howe, entrepreneur and founder, USA*

This is not just a stirring, motivational but ultimately hollow speech that will turn out to be 100 per cent untrue when you get out there and start pursuing your career dreams. Thanks to countless campaigners that went before us (see, I told you us Type 1s are a formidable lot!), it is now illegal in the UK and many other places for employers to discriminate against, or even exclude, anyone with diabetes. There are, I will add, a handful of exceptions. The armed forces have a blanket ban on anyone with the condition and certain emergency services also have rules about diabetics applying for jobs. The same goes for airlines and air traffic control, which are exempt from disability discrimination laws. There are regional variations to what some services will allow, so if you are hell bent on a career in this direction, you should do some digging. Expect some rigorous assessments and medical evaluations if you decide to pursue a career in any of these areas.

WHAT YOU SAY ABOUT TYPE 1 IS UP TO YOU

When you begin to apply for jobs, one of the first things to realise is that it is up to you how much, or how little, you speak about Type 1. For most jobs, there is no obligation to say anything about it at all and it is, in fact, illegal for your employer to ask questions about it to assess your suitability for the job in relation to your condition. I say 'most jobs'. Even some of the less physically demanding professions do have special requirements where employers will have to decide whether or not your condition could prevent you from carrying out the role, or if any adjustments needed to help you do so are not possible. In these cases, expect health questions to be raised at the application stage.

Even if you don't *have* to declare your Type 1 in your application, you might feel that it makes good sense to tell your would-be employer. It won't make you less likely to get the job (because they can't legally use this information against you) but, if you highlight it from the off, it shows that you are positive about your condition and organised in managing it. It could even boost your application since many organisations have pledged to increase the representation of disabled people in their ranks and are predisposed to look upon applications from people with conditions favourably.

I'm a category manager for frozen food at a Swedish retailer that sells a range of foods such as fruits, vegetables, seafood, meat, bread and pasta, with a focus on health. I said I had Type 1 when they hired me. For me it was important because I wanted them to know what the reason would be if I needed to take a few days off, for example to deliver a speech somewhere.

My colleagues don't react in any specific way. They ask if they are curious about something but, in the main, they don't care. And I like that I am a 'normal' person to them. Sometimes I need to eat during meetings because of low blood sugar. Occasionally people react and ask questions but this barely ever happens.

Sara Mobäck, influencer, Sweden

WORK ISSUES? THERE'S ALWAYS A SOLUTION

You may be wondering whether or not you will need to choose between highly physical or less rigorous office work. As mentioned, my first paid job was in a high-volume, fast-paced French restaurant. My main duty there was to deliver food from the kitchen to the dining area. The task generally involved multiple dishes, laden on a heavy tray, all weighing up to 12–15 kg. That in itself felt like an upper-body workout for my 50 kg self. Meanwhile, those trays needed to be carried gracefully (it was a *fine* French restaurant) and we were also responsible for making sure every item was clean and tidy, matching the restaurant's exacting standards. Oh, and we needed to add coffee-making to our skill set too. Now, this was not a small kitchen and the step count on my iPhone often equalled what I'd do on my 18-hole golf games! There wasn't a big difference between this experience and my early experiences with sports. I just needed to work out the best way of doing it, for my needs.

I didn't have my continuous glucose monitoring (CGM) device when I first joined the restaurant. Foolishly, I took the attitude that I'd been doing sports my entire life so it would be easy. As it turned out, it was not as straightforward as I envisaged. I found myself taking more breaks than my colleagues thanks to the constant blood glucose checks required. The workload was unpredictable, so it wasn't easy to stick to a schedule and manage it appropriately. But there's always a solution, right? That's when I got the CGM. There was only one more hurdle to jump after that. We were not allowed to have our phones with us while we were working, and yet I needed my phone to be able to check my CGM reading. Again, there was a solution. I spoke to the restaurant management, explained my issue and made them a compelling offer. If they let me keep my phone with me (for CGM checks only), I would need considerably fewer breaks and would therefore work far more efficiently. They agreed and all my problems disappeared in an instant. Blood glucose uncertainty was no longer an issue and didn't disturb me when I was completing my duties (and getting a full-body workout with those heavy trays!).

In recent years, I've also had the chance to experience office life. Indeed, I am still experiencing it while part of Cass Business School's accelerator with my start-up (see chapter four). There is much less physical action in an office and a lot more thinking going on. But, this doesn't mean blood glucose levels can be ignored. I know that I can rarely think and concentrate when my levels start on a roller-coaster-like journey, so I carefully schedule activities outside work (those morning runs in chapter five!) that make blood glucose management easier and improve my daytime concentration. This also means that the ever-present office cakes, biscuits and sweets are more easily ignored. I say *more easily* ignored, but it is not always possible to avoid the temptations!

Bar the exceptions listed earlier, the sky is the limit when you are weighing up what to do as a career. In fact, while discussing professions with Matt Collins for this book, we considered the question of whether or not there are any professions we physically couldn't do. The only one we could really think of was becoming an astronaut. Once we'd finished our conversation, a sceptical voice inside me made me reach for my laptop and search for 'diabetic astronauts' on the web. Guess what? This is how I discovered that even the sky is not the limit for our Type 1 astronaut Josu Feijoo!

I absolutely think that my diabetes influenced my decision to study to be a PE teacher. When I was 17 years old, I began to work out more and realised that me and my diabetes felt better because of that. Thanks to my diabetes community in Sweden, I got the opportunity to climb the highest mountain in the country in 2017. That experience was also the start of a more adventurous life for me, and I think that was a big influence on my career decision.

Elin Sandström, health and PE student and influencer, Sweden

Your own career choice depends entirely on what you want to do and what you feel best suits your interests, skills and needs. You may, for example, be more comfortable with a job that requires you to do regular physical exercise, rather than one where you'd be sitting behind a desk all day. Alternatively, the routine of an office job may be exactly what you crave. It's entirely up to you.

Something to consider is the hours you'll be working and whether or not they'll be on a shift basis. When I started working at the restaurant, going through a 11am–11pm shift one day and then switching to 7am–3pm on another day and then over to 3pm–2am was a new experience for me. In fact, the timetable allocation reminded me of gambling in a casino. Every week the waiting staff would be presented with a schedule for the following week and the management seemed keen to ensure that we didn't ever feel like we were in a repetitive routine! Shift work can be really handy for someone who hates routine, but it does require management. You certainly need to make sure you are good with adjusting your blood glucose to fit your daily schedule. I admire anyone with the discipline to manage this well, I must admit!

Working 9 to 5 (or whatever your x to y is) daily makes for great general day planning. It is handy to know when you start and when you finish, even if office life doesn't always mean you experience the same thing day in, day out. There will always be cases of overrun meetings, which can potentially lead to a late lunch or rescheduled activities.

Going it alone and being your own boss is also a very viable option. Many contributors to this book have chosen this path. My personal favourite advantage of this option is that if there are occasional periods when your blood glucose is raging, it is possible to take a one- or two-

Yes, you can!

hour break to even things out. Ditto if you'd like to schedule any physical activities. You can always finish the required task later and there is no need to explain anything to management.

> My life changed a lot after I was diagnosed. The most significant way was my career choice. I went from wanting to be a hip-hop music producer to being someone who performs work associated with nutrition and diabetes. This is mainly because I became way more health conscious than I was before. I became aware of my food intake and the carbohydrates I was eating, and I started exercising anywhere from three to six times a week.
>
> With diabetes as my main focus, I wanted to help other people living with diabetes. This meant always practising what I preached: positivity towards diabetes and living a healthy life.
>
> Today, I work with special needs adults as a part-time job coach for what is called a 'partial day programme', from 8am to 2pm. If I am not doing that, I am usually working out, eating or cooking. Then, my main passion is creating diabetic content on social media, which might be editing podcasts (the podcast I co-host is called *Pardon my Pancreas*) or creating some content for my own Instagram page, and I used to do daily vlogs too.
>
> *Ali Abdulkareem, blogger and job coach, USA*

TELLING YOUR COLLEAGUES ABOUT TYPE 1

Do you tell your closest co-workers about your Type 1? It's completely up to you. My suggestions would be very similar to those in chapter two (on telling others). You can make up your mind when and what to say. Most of the time, people will either be very curious or completely oblivious. While having lunch in the office one time, a colleague asked me if he could borrow a pen. Of course, I agreed straight away. Yet, while I was searching for one in my bag, I noticed that the person had already found one and was sauntering away, back to his desk. Except, he hadn't found any old pen. He'd found my insulin pen. Naturally, he had no clue that it was anything other than a writing device. The look of surprise on his face when he sat down and opened the pen will stay with me forever.

On another afternoon, I spotted *my pen* lying on someone else's desk. There are a lot of start-ups in the place where I work, with people from different teams minding their own business (hehe). 'Ahh great, someone else has decided to borrow a pen,' I thought. I walked over to the desk to retrieve it and then got on with my work. Half an hour later, I became aware of a guy running around the office, desperately searching for something. It wasn't long before he raised his voice and asked the magic question, 'Has anyone seen my insulin pen?' Silence. 'It looks like an oversized writing pen,' he explained. I picked up the pen and held it aloft so he could see it, all the while wondering how I was going to explain why I had taken his insulin pen. We laughed about it afterwards and compared notes. It was, in fact, this person who was the first to show me a real, live CGM. As it happened, this was exactly when I was figuring my blood glucose levels out in relation to the restaurant schedule. It was what finally convinced me to look seriously at getting a CGM. What a lifechanging experience pen-borrowing is, I have to say.

> I was working up in London, about an hour's train ride from my home in Kent, when I first got diagnosed. I'd then need to walk another half an hour to get to the office and the same in reverse after eight to ten hours in the office. It wasn't a particular challenge. I'd check my blood before I got on the train and then just before I got off. I'd do the same when I left the office. It is just a sensible precaution. It's no different from any other sort of preparation when you get into a routine.
>
> The people I work with closely know about my Type 1 and that helps. If they see me acting slightly strangely, they say, 'Do you want to get your sugar or something?' Obviously, it is up to you who you tell. I wouldn't necessarily tell a new client that 'by the way, I have diabetes'. They just don't need to know. I would if I am going to be working with them for any period of time, or if I am in and out of their offices. That just seems sensible. If they know in advance, it'll prevent a lot of worrying should any unforeseen circumstances happen.
>
> *Kevin Stewart, publishing contracts consultant, UK*

Yes, you can!

Telling your colleagues that you have diabetes can create a kind of team spirit, especially when you have a common goal to work towards. As long as you are engaged and prove to be a valuable part of the team, everyone will be eager to help out at any moment.

> I've been hypo on air a fair few times and it's just been a real struggle to get through. But then, I'm in the studio environment, so that's fine. The weirdest thing that happened to me was when I was hosting a conference for the UK's deputy prime minister about ten years ago. I was so hypo when I got up on the stage to close the conference that I really cannot remember what I said. I think that I was probably talking gibberish and that it was awful, really awful. I was absolutely mortified.
>
> I think that if it happened today, I would just say, 'I need to get a coke or something. I'm really sorry, I'm Type 1 and I'm going really hypo. I need to take five minutes.' You definitely get a bit bolder as you get older. It would have been embarrassing but it would have been a lot better. But, instead, I just tried to carry on and it just got worse and worse and worse.
>
> *Stephen Dixon, Sky News presenter, UK*

As with any career, there are no promises that everything will always go to plan, but what ever does? Just do what you do, enjoy the good times, develop a sense of humour about the bad ones and you'll amazed about what you can achieve.

> I really didn't know what I wanted to do after school. I wanted to do something related to diabetes, but I didn't know what. I thought it might be to become a doctor or nurse and did start out as a pre-med student, but I wasn't really happy there. I didn't feel like that was for me at all. So, I thought again. Ever since I was a child, I had always been into art and design, but I never really explored graphic design. After taking a few classes in that programme, I decided to change and get a degree in graphic design. For the last three and a half years, I have really taken

that programme into my life. In the last year I created a whole body of work that is diabetes related, in the form of graphic design. Now, with my degree in this field, I want to further my education and become a Certified Diabetes Educator. I will combine diabetes and graphic design into a career somehow.

David Mina, graphic designer, USA

8

NIGHTS OUT WITH FRIENDS

Yes, you can!

The first time I met someone 'in the wild' with diabetes was pretty funny. I was in line at Chipotle, the Mexican fast-food place, and this guy walked by and saw my pump tubing. Out of nowhere, he said, 'Yo! Me too!' and showed me his pump. That was it. Then he just walked on. He was such a funny, energetic dude. I'll never forget it.

Rob Howe, entrepreneur and founder, USA

Up until I was 15 years old, my visits to restaurants and public places looked something like this (especially when I was going out with people I didn't know too well):

- Check my blood glucose before I arrive.
- Meet the others while outwardly steadfastly paying no attention to my blood sugar.
- Inwardly, begin trying to predict the trends in my blood glucose (while effecting the look of not looking at all concerned).
- Even when everyone orders something to share that I know is not good for me, don't inject, because of not wanting to make anyone uncomfortable.

It wasn't a great situation – not least because how can anyone really relax when, at the back of their mind, there is a niggling suspicion that their lovely convivial evening won't end well? By behaving like this, the chances were quite high that I would have a hypo, or at least have a few 'interesting' hours struggling with soaring blood glucose levels.

There were times in my life where I cared a lot what other people thought of me with diabetes, but all it did was take up precious mental space. Now I live my life and do what I have to do, but if someone ever stops me to ask what my insulin pump is, I'll gladly take the time to stop and explain to them. I've found that in these interactions it's mostly curiosity over anything else.

Lauren Bongiorno, diabetes health coach, USA

Nights Out With Friends

Like Lauren, I too am a lot different today, and far more confident, but I also recognise that it has taken me time to get there. Socialising can seem like a bit of a minefield for anyone with Type 1, especially the newly diagnosed. Family and close friends will be considerate and understanding, but what happens when you are with people you don't know all that well? Also, how will strangers react if they see you injecting? When you go out with friends, alcohol and sometimes even drugs may be on the agenda. There are often social pressures to join in and be 'one of the guys', but the future implications for anyone with diabetes are potentially far graver than a sore head or doing a few daft things.

TREATING BLOOD GLUCOSE PUBLICLY

Let's start with the issue that will most likely be uppermost in anyone's mind: injections. Mindset is very important here. There is *nothing wrong* with having diabetes. It is easy to say, but it's true. It is what it is, as they say, so manage it, be proud of who you are and use it to spur you on to ever greater things. Injections are just part of managing your life.

After a brief period when I lacked in confidence, I have reached a stage where I really don't care about where I inject. I find the most suitable location in the circumstance and do what I need to do. We do it because for us it's like breathing – we just have to.

> When I was on pens, I thought there was always a slightly strange reaction. Even when I used a blood glucose meter, people were quite taken aback when they saw it. I never went to the bathroom and hid away, though. I always did it in public, to make a point, I think. Now, I'm on a pump and I use CGM (continuous glucose monitoring device), so most of the time there's no visible thing to anybody. Although I quite like the fact that with CGM, I have this sensor on my arm, so if I'm in a t-shirt, people can see it and ask about it. I quite like being able to show it off a little bit, rather than hide it away.
>
> *Stephen Dixon, Sky News presenter, UK*

Yes, you can!

SOCIAL PLANNING

Whenever I socialise, I make sure to spend some time preparing. How long I spend usually depends on the type of event. Experience has shown me that there is a significant difference between having a simple dinner that will last a couple of hours and a more ambitious evening where I will perhaps eat and then go on somewhere else to dance and hang out. Either way, having diabetes doesn't mean you shouldn't enjoy yourself just as much as everyone else.

The easiest scenario is hosting a dinner at home. This way you are calling the shots. Often your guests will offer to bring something along but this is your opportunity to give them the chance to enjoy some of your favourite (and carb familiar!) dishes. Healthy eating isn't just for Type 1s.

If you are meeting everyone at a restaurant or café, forewarned is forearmed. Most eating places are online these days, so check the menu ahead of time so you know what to expect. Scope out the healthy balanced choices and plan your meal in an unhurried fashion. I try to order food with a predictable carb count so I know exactly how much I need to inject. If that is not entirely possible, some sure trips and tricks are substituting fries with a salad or steamed vegetables, or enjoying your burger without the carb-heavy bun. The point of a bit of prior research is to take the guesswork out of ordering later on, so you can relax and enjoy time with your friends. Once again, I would just like to clarify something here: I'm not suggesting that you can't eat any of these things. You can! It is simply easier to control social interactions when we are aware of the carbs we eat. To completely relax and enjoy your downtime, stick to more familiar and transparent carb counts.

Before you head out of the door, check your blood glucose levels. This won't be the only time you do this throughout the evening, though. No matter where you are going or what you are doing, always keep track, just as you would whether or not you are socialising. This is a lot easier today with CGMs, which measure levels in real time without you having to think about it. Just make a discrete check on your smartphone, which is what everyone else will be doing all the time anyhow. (Well, not checking their blood glucose, but certainly keeping an eye on their messages.)

A 'LOW BLOOD GLUCOSE GUIDE' FOR FRIENDS

While discretion is great, it's helpful if at least one other person in the group is aware of your Type 1. They can keep an eye out for you and take action if you experience a high or low. So, what exactly should you be saying to your close buddies? Well, if they see you, or any other diabetic friend, sweating, going pale, appearing confused and speaking nonsense, they should say, 'Check your blood sugar!' If it is really low (below 4 mmol/L (72 mg/dL)), they should feed you with 15–20 g of fast-acting glucose. Anything like a sugary drink, fizzy drinks (not the 'sugar-free' or 'zero' alternatives, please!), fruit juice or sugar drops is good. They should also always ask you to sit down, because if the condition persists and the sweets don't work immediately, there is a risk you may fall over, or worse still go into a coma.

Tell them it is very *unlikely* to happen, but if you do go into coma, they should immediately:

1. Ascertain the reason for the coma, which could be because of low (not high) blood sugar. This means checking your blood glucose.
2. If your blood sugar is low, take your glucagon (glycogen) pen and inject it into your arms or legs.
3. If you don't wake up within 15 minutes, call an ambulance.

The good news is, such events are very rare – so rare I've never had one in 20 years. And they can be prevented with even the slightest degree of care and attention. However, if there is any uncertainty, it is better to call an ambulance immediately and treat the situation as an emergency.

> I suppose I was a bit uncomfortable about my diabetes to begin with. I remember quite a few occasions when I was at university, wandering around being really hypo and not daring tell anybody that I needed to go and get some chocolate or anything. Now, I don't know really why that was. Now it's fine, and that's partly because of the job. I sort of feel I have a responsibility, being in the public eye, to be open about it. I want to help other people and it's a very rewarding thing to be able to do so.
>
> *Stephen Dixon, Sky News presenter, UK*

Yes, you can!

CARRYING SUPPLIES (PENS AND WATER)

Carrying around pens (if you use them) will quickly become second nature. But make sure that you don't forget them in the excitement of getting dressed up. You will also need to get used to carting around water. People tend to make funny comments about my thirst for water, but honestly, I don't think I can ever have too much of it. On average, I drink four litres of water a day. When somebody makes a comment or gives me a surprised look, I tend to reply with the words of my endocrinologist: water helps to regulate your temperature, lubricate your joints and get rid of waste. Also, many of us often mistake feeling thirsty for feeling hungry. If you think you feel hungry, try a glass of water first, especially if your blood glucose is high. It'll stop you over-eating.

I never go *anywhere* without my trusty 1.5-litre water bottle – cafés, dining places, cinemas, museums, everywhere. For environmentally conscious people, carrying their own water containers seems absolutely normal behaviour. However, others do get surprised by the constant presence of my water bottle, although most people are more curious about the fact that I can drink that much in one sitting. I do also find myself being judged for bringing my own bottle to venues such as restaurants where it is not necessary the norm. It's usually just a raised eyebrow though, and anyone who does ask is generally very understanding when I tell them why. How could they not be?

ALCOHOL AND DEHYDRATION

Nights out are the time when alcohol flows freely and, depending upon your social set, there is occasionally some pressure to imbibe. Personally, I've never been a big drinker. Alcohol can have a big impact on your health over and above the usual warnings about sticking to recommended amounts. When you drink, less water is reabsorbed into the kidneys and more goes to the bladder, which is why people need to go to the loo more when they drink. With less water being retained, we're far more likely to become dehydrated – which is exactly what you are working against by carrying around that water bottle. You may think you are taking on a lot of water, but when you drink, you'll excrete a great deal of your good efforts. The effects of a 'good session' don't end when you say goodbye to everyone either. Alcohol can lead to a lowering of blood glucose levels overnight.

Nights Out With Friends

The big thing to say here is: we are all different and react to alcohol differently. Let me share with you my first big experience of drinking a cocktail containing strong spirits to illustrate this. I had heard more than a few horror stories from other diabetics about how strong alcohol took their blood glucose down during a night out, which was partly why I'd never tried it. On the day of my graduation ball from school, I decided the time had come to experiment. And what wonders! I took things very easy, but I didn't experience any unusual blood glucose reaction on the night. I was overjoyed and had a great time with my classmates too.

The sense of self-satisfaction lasted until the next morning. I woke up, injected and ate as usual, and then, out of nowhere, suddenly experienced a very unexpected, true hypo. My blood glucose would not go up for the entire day, even though, except for the morning injection, I didn't treat any of my meals with insulin. All this from one cocktail! Then, the next morning, I found my blood glucose in the skies.

All in all, it was not a good experiment. After I got everything back under control and had time to reflect, I concluded that everybody's blood glucose reacts differently to alcohol. Even so, I decided to give it a second chance a year later. And guess what? The effect was the same. Wasn't it Einstein who said the definition of insanity is doing the same thing over and over and expecting a different result? So, what did I learn from this? I confirmed that my body has a late reaction to alcohol. Since then, I have reduced my consumption to the very minimum, and only the very lightest versions of drinks. I don't really mind since I have never felt it necessary to drink to have fun and personally don't feel anyone of any age should drink too much, but each to their own. To drink socially, Type 1s need to be aware of how their bodies respond to alcohol in order to keep everything under control, adjust insulin when needed and stay safe.

I should also add, I have just as much fun, maybe more, when I don't drink. Once, when my blood glucose went extremely low in a club, I ordered a simple orange juice at the bar to urgently get my blood glucose up. The barman only had a vodka-orange glass, so he used that. I swigged the 100 per cent orange juice all in one go – there's no hesitation when blood glucose is low. But it was so low that I needed a second glass. Again, I knocked back the glass in one go, which surprised the barman a little. Then, when I got back to normal again, I caught the surprised stare of two chaps who'd observed the entire scene of me downing two glasses of

Yes, you can!

'vodka-orange' in quick succession. They simply commented, 'Impressive!' They thought the glasses had been full of alcohol. I laughed, thanked them and joined my friends on the dancefloor with renewed energy.

Unusual? Maybe, but that's how we can best enjoy our dancing and fun time with friends.

> On one night out, drinking with a friend of mine, I decided to be a very good boy. I thought, 'I'm going to drink alcohol-free beer tonight!' Of course, well, I completely forgot that alcohol free doesn't mean 'sugar free'. Frankly, it means the opposite.
>
> The next day my sugar was sky high because I forgot that my drinks were basically just full of sugar and I hadn't taken any extra injections. I never made that mistake again.
>
> Diabetes is all about learning and it is OK to make mistakes. It's about learning about yourself, your body, about the things that you're putting into your body. It's hard to tell someone in a similar position what to do, because everybody's body reacts in a different way to so many things.
>
> *Kevin Stewart, publishing contracts consultant, UK*

Whenever I've been given a challenge along the lines of 'drink or we don't respect you', 'drink or you don't belong in the group' or any other variation designed to oblige me to drink alcohol, I have always turned down the offer and known that I would not go out with that group again. Most people respect my choice, though, just as I have respected theirs. That's the freedom you should have. No one has to give in to this peer pressure (whether or not we have Type 1) and if you are with a group that doesn't get this, maybe you're in the wrong group. But hey, in order to understand where we belong, we also need to understand where we don't belong.

None of this means you can flat-out never drink at all. However, do check ahead with your healthcare team to see whether or not you are able to drink. Alcohol reacts badly with some medication. Even if you are given the green light to drink, you should certainly always eat food when drinking, to help keep your blood sugar levels steady. And don't forget to keep checking your blood glucose levels. It's easy to relax when you are feeling mellow and this is the time you really need to be on the ball.

If you do find yourself overdoing it, don't get upset. We all do it. It's a learning experience. Be sure to test your blood glucose levels in the morning, since the symptoms of a hangover (such as headaches, feeling sick, sweating and shaking) are similar to those you get with a hypo. Don't be tempted to skip meals to 'get yourself back on track' – you'll only end up over-eating on the next meal, which could in turn cause high blood sugar. Always have breakfast the morning after the night before, even if you don't feel like it. Get back to your daily schedule as soon as you can (hangover notwithstanding), test your blood glucose levels often, take your meds and you'll be back to your usual lovely, healthy self in no time.

RETAINING JUDGEMENT

Your favoured tipple is entirely up to you, but you're better off sticking to dry wine or Prosecco, which have a relatively low carb count compared to super-sugary drinks like alcopops. If you must have spirits, stick to the diet versions of mixers (that's where the 'sugar-free' and 'zero' alternatives become handy!). Whatever you drink, pace yourself and alternate any drink with a glass of water, which gives your body a chance to metabolise the alcohol. If you are somewhere like a nightclub, where food is generally not readily available but you know you'll be drinking, carry some snacks with you.

Try to retain some level of judgement, which is not always easy after a drink. The main causes of hypos are an overdose of insulin (where the person with Type 1 hasn't eaten enough food), exercise or too much alcohol. A combination of all of the above is the highest-risk scenario. This is why preparation and planning are so important. If, for example, your big night out is likely to end in some dancing, or better still a lot of dancing, keep a very close eye on your levels. Dancing is exercise and, for some people, pretty energetic exercise. Ditto, if you are walking from venue to venue, you'd be surprised at how much distance you cover. The combined effect really drags your blood glucose down. To make matters worse, the first signs of a hypo are not unlike feeling tipsy, so they often go neglected. Thus, anyone going on a night out where food and drink are involved should be sure there is at least one, if not more, person who is aware of the right treatment for a hypo.

The most common error of judgement in this scenario is forgetting whether you have injected or not. This has happened to me, and I can still remember the feeling of confusion as I stood in my room, concentrating and staring at my basal (night-time) pen. *Have I injected or have I not?* It was the first time in my life that I'd forgotten whether I'd injected my night-time basal, and it happened after a great evening of dancing and having fun with my friends.

There are few moments that are truly dangerous for a diabetic. This is certainly one of them. The wrong answer will ruin all the plans you've got for the next 24 hours. Injecting basal insulin twice might result in a rapid night-time hypo, giving you no time to react, and you will find yourself in hypos for a day. But, if you inject nothing at all, you will have to deal with high blood glucose for 24 hours. It's almost like gambling.

So, had I injected or not?

I decided *not* to inject. It was what my intuition and common sense told me, and it is commonly believed to be the safer option. In situations like this, high blood glucose levels are safer than hypos. After that, I went to sleep.

Waking up at 7am, I could feel my heart pumping as my blood glucose decided to shake up my morning by skyrocketing from 5.3 to 17.0 mmol/L (95 to 306 mg/dL) within 30 minutes. It kept up the same trend throughout the day.

Turns out I had taken the wrong bet by deciding not to inject anything. It was the first time in my life – and I hope will be the last time – when I forgot to inject my basal. It was a great lesson though. Since then, I have prepared seven needles for the week ahead every Sunday, and change one after each injection. If I get hesitant, I simply re-count how many days and needles are left for the week, and know instantly if I have injected or not.

Injecting is very routine, but when you do it every single day of the year for several years, you can easily find yourself unsure about whether the injection you remember happened today or yesterday. My strong advice is to find your way to let yourself know if you've injected. It's very handy, especially after days when you've let your discipline off the hook for a bit.

Remember: a bit of planning and preparation does not make you the odd one out. Your mates will all prepare for a big night out in a largely similar fashion. They'll have a few drinks, a bit of a boogie, maybe some chips on the way home and a large glass of water before bed. You're doing pretty much the same thing, but just on a more measured basis!

SOME NOTES ON DRUGS

The other reality of a night out these days is that drugs are often on offer. I am not interested myself, but I do know others are and I am not here to judge. If you are tempted, the same guidelines apply for drugs as they do for alcohol: use your judgement. Even small amounts of drugs can have an impact on your blood glucose levels, not least because all the usual routines go out of the window. Some drugs will slow you down, while others will give you more energy: the obvious impact is that your blood glucose levels will soar or sink. In what could be a perfect storm, you may lose track of time and become relaxed about checking your blood glucose levels, or forget to eat or take your insulin. Equally worrying, the effects of the drugs may disguise the warning signs of an impending hypo. The effects last too. You may experience a 'come down' for at least a couple of days afterwards, which can affect your mood and your ability to look after yourself and manage your diabetes. If you still feel you want to dabble with drugs, it is worth having a conversation with your healthcare team, who can offer you some advice and guidance. If you don't feel able to do this, at the very least make sure you are with a good friend who agrees not to take drugs, who knows about your diabetes and who knows how to recognise and help you treat a hypo.

There has been very little research about the effects of recreational drugs on those with diabetes. If you decide you want to partake, this is something you will need to find out for yourself (while taking great care, please!). One resource you might consider is reaching out to others in the diabetic community. We are an incredible bunch and, as I have discovered, are very willing to help and advise one another. Whether it is drugs, exercise or how to deal with a particular diabetes-related issue with work, friends or your home life, there is someone, somewhere who has gone through something similar and who can offer valuable advice and counsel.

'HEY, ME TOO!'

As a teenager, I did occasionally feel like an outcast because I never met anyone outside hospital with Type 1 diabetes. I had a strong need to be accepted as part of a group of like-minded people. I didn't mention this to my friendship group and it didn't really occur to me to reach out further afield. It was only when I began my research for this book that

Yes, you can!

I realised that there is a wonderful community out there. We don't just share a condition, either: we share a strong desire to help one another. I have developed a huge sense of belonging. The people I meet, mainly online, live through the same experiences as me and totally understand all the issues that bug me.

I mention this here, in a chapter on socialising, for two reasons. The first reason is that your diabetic peers are a rich source of advice and help on all issues about your condition, going out and having fun. And, second, it's fun to socialise with people from this community! I am in touch with people who have Type 1 from around the world and I love it. I can't tell you the number of times I have practically yelled 'Hey, me too!' at my computer screen. Thanks to this incredible online community, I have, for the first time in my life, encountered a huge dose of pride about having the 'disease'. I also feel an abundance of love and solidarity towards everyone who has it. Collectively, they've made me want to show that I am proud too! I'm happy to show off this cool thing I have. In fact, it was this incredible bunch that helped me to finally decide to get a CGM.

Don't just take my word for it. Reach out. I've included a number of websites you may like to look up in the appendix. You will find that the people behind them are inspiring and motivating. They will help you find the courage to show off the condition that makes *our community* special. We learn a lot from each other on a daily basis. Our interactions not only help us to feel understood but are also a source of hands-on tips and tricks that can help you manage whatever issue you face. Take my advice: widen your social circle and get online.

Social media is a great place to gather information, find answers to some questions that might be bothering you and find your community. Like with anything on social media, you should be very selective on whom to follow and whom to place as your role model – especially if you want to make treatment decisions based on the person's advice. Overall, though, it is terrific to see how the conversation around diabetes has progressed from a rare topic to an ongoing discussion. It is very exciting to see where it all goes.

It's good to have a like-minded community, even though

I've always felt super-comfortable with diabetes and with saying out loud that I have Type 1 diabetes, or showing off diabetes supplies. I am lucky because I have always had very understanding friends. How people elsewhere have reacted has always been a matter of location. Some places, people are more conservative about it than in others. I once had a date with a girl and, when I took out my insulin pen, she said, 'This is disgusting, go to the bathroom and do it there.' I was a bit mystified by that. From my perspective, the bathroom is the dirtiest place in the entire building! Why would I do it there?!

Matt Collins, robotic surgery business leader, USA

RELATIONSHIPS

Ah yes, relationships. How could I conclude a chapter on socialising without exploring one of the most crucial aspects of our social lives? Relationships are something that everyone with Type 1 will inevitably give a lot of thought to, sooner or later. Meeting, and getting to know, a potential partner is daunting enough without wondering when, where and how you introduce the rather important matter of your diabetes. First-date nerves can be bad, but this could pitch you into unknown and stressful territory.

Speak to any person in the same position and you'll quickly discover that one way most people try to get through the dating minefield is humour (which, come to think of it, isn't bad advice for anyone, whether or not they have diabetes). Stories abound of insulin pump tangles, hypos at *exactly* the wrong moment (definitely a bit of a passion killer) and well-made plans ditched in favour of a mad dash to get insulin.

But, let's begin at the beginning. When do you broach the subject? It might be tempting to get it out of the way as soon as possible, but that is a big load of stress to add to an already awkward social situation. You may be better off treating it like you would on any other night out with a new crowd – only mention it when it comes up. Don't make a big thing out of it. I've learned that if I am calm and casual about it, so are the people I tell. Treat it as a big story and others will react in exactly the same way. Speak of it as a burden and so will they. And so on! So, as they say, 'Smart casual is the sure way!' This will make it seem like no big deal, which of course it isn't. You'll most likely find your date will know quite a lot about

Yes, you can!

it anyway, since there are plenty of people around with diabetes these days. You could use the opportunity to dispel a few myths too.

Another huge problem that I observe is fear among girls when it comes to telling their boyfriends that they have diabetes. I was afraid to do this too, so I know it can be hard. Then, I met someone and, after a week or two of dating, I admitted to him that I had the condition. He surprised me by saying he knew everything about it! Now, I am sure that if a person loves you, they will care about your wellbeing and won't be scared of any condition you might have. Oh, and after about one and a half years with this guy, we got married. Today, we are a happy family that's been together for five years and it is totally wonderful.

It is very important not to hide your diabetes and not to hide yourself. If you do, it will be much harder to explain later on in the relationship.

Kornelia Mango, singer and celebrity, Russia

The other big hurdle to cross is injecting for the first time in front of your new partner. You never know in advance if they are going to be incredibly squeamish or just curious. Again, it's best not to force the issue by waving supplies in front of their face! Be as discrete as you would be with any new crowd. If they are cool with learning more or being more involved, they can ask. If they make a huge deal about it – or tell you it's disgusting, like Mike's date did – there is a chance that this person is probably not the best boyfriend or girlfriend material for you. It's their loss. They'll never get to learn what an incredible person you are.

If your dates go well and the relationship gets physical, there is no reason why you shouldn't enjoy your sex life as much as anyone else, bearing in mind all the same provisos, such as using protection. The only difference to remember is that this activity constitutes exercise, so you will need to follow all the guidance about that.

Nights Out With Friends

I've had some uncomfortable moments when dating guys. Once, I didn't tell a guy I was dating that I had diabetes, then he found out and his reaction was, 'Why didn't you tell me you have diabetes?' I told him that I was afraid he was going to reject me. But, he told me that I was silly. 'I would never reject you for this.'

In Sweden, the people I meet are very open about diabetes. But there are groups that are shy, who hide away and are ashamed of themselves. I accept that there are sometimes horrible comments made in restaurants and in public, but my view is we need to show the rest of the world *our reality*. I want to live. I need to survive. Injections are my survival kit, so I can't bother caring about what other people think!

Sara Mobäck, influencer, Sweden

One last, but not least, important note. We can have a healthy child. As you'd possibly imagine, pregnancy brings with it a need for extra care for women with diabetes, including more visits to doctors and additional health check-ups. However, with the careful observation of doctors, it is all possible. I can't present my personal experience on this yet; however, I am absolutely confident my moment of motherhood will come and am looking forward to this time of my life with much anticipation.

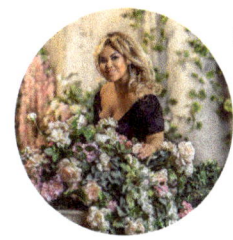

I would like to become a mum! I dream of having children. In fact, if I was entirely honest, I'd say my desires to be a mum (and a good wife) and to give birth to healthy kids are my main motivations to keep my sugars stable.

Kornelia Mango, singer and celebrity, Russia

9

MIND, BODY AND SOUL: HAVING DIABETES UNDER CONTROL, MENTALLY, PHYSICALLY AND EMOTIONALLY

Yes, you can!

I have been living with Type 1 diabetes since I was 7 years old and, today, I am an online diabetic health coach and the creator of *The Diabetic Health Journal*. Diabetes set the stage for me to really get to know myself on a deep, deep level. I don't think that everyone with diabetes can necessarily say that, but the opportunity is there for all of us and it's up to us to take it or not. At this point in my life, I truly love learning from my habits, thoughts and behaviours, and watching as I make the connections between what serves me and what does not, on all different levels, whether it is blood sugars, food, relationships, places or people.

I wouldn't say my life is all about diabetes, but it does play a large role. My life is about love, passion, happiness, feeling confident in my own skin and impacting other people's lives. But these things are not accessible to me if I don't feel good on a daily basis. And much of how I feel on a daily basis, whether that be my mood or energy levels, is dependent upon my blood sugars.

Most people, when they are newly diagnosed, don't receive the resources they need on a holistic level to better understand how their bodies work and to feel like they are in control. A dream of mine is to see more of a bridge between hospitals and outside resources. I strongly believe that until there is a cure, we need to take control of our diabetes, and for most of us that means having the proper support, guidance and accountability to do so. This is why I coach and create resources for people with diabetes all over the world, to help them achieve optimal diabetes management and feel strong and empowered. My practice is rooted in a 360-degree approach, emphasising wellness throughout the mind, body and soul. I believe that through self-reflection and mindfulness we are better able to understand our own patterns, achieve our goals and reform our most limiting habits.

Lauren Bongiorno, diabetes health coach, USA

You are limitless. You can climb mountains, embark on your favourite career, become the next have-to-see celebrity or save other people's lives.

We don't just control what we choose to do either. We can also control the fact that we're happy while we do it. Yet, our limitless opportunities only exist if we have diabetes under control, as much as that is in our hands. If you know anything about trading on the stock market, you'll realise that the principle is similar: patience is key, even when things go very well. Impulsive reactions to fluctuations are never a winning strategy, even when they are the most intuitive thing to do. If you give way to these impulses, the consequences can be expensive. Our expense is our health, not cash, though, so it is in our interest to learn how to be attentive, patient and disciplined – and, very importantly, retain our sense of humour. This way we can seamlessly manage our blood glucose levels while embarking on life's adventures.

SELF-AWARENESS

Self-awareness is your friend when it comes to controlling Type 1. By this I mean being aware of your moment-by-moment thoughts, emotions and physical sensations, in a non-judgemental way. This is pretty valuable in diabetes management because it helps you understand what is happening to your body and when, so you can react on time to stay in control.

I didn't think much about this process in my early years, but now I have learned more about it, I realise that I have been (albeit unwittingly) doing it for a while and that I find it very useful. To show how, let me explain the three-stage process I go through when my blood sugar gets low.

Stage 1: Fun. The very first sign my blood sugar is sinking is when I start to make the most awful, awful jokes. Seriously, I mean quips that would make even the most jovial group groan in exasperation. The jokes are so bad, they are actually funny. At least that is what I hear from my friends, who seem to enjoy this stage a lot. Take away the humour (and yes, I know everyone would be pleased if I did!) and just below it is a rapturous feeling of 100 per cent happiness. This is the time, more than any other, when I feel inspired. Inside my head, I am a genius. I could solve the toughest maths puzzle, negotiate world peace, paint the most extraordinary artwork, anything! I am so in the moment and fully aware of everything around me, it is as if a whole new sense has opened up. I often wonder whether this is what healthy people always feel like. If so: lucky them! *They are blessed.*

Yes, you can!

Stage 2: Drunk. OK, not properly drunk, but I feel like it and I display all the tell-tale symptoms of overdoing it on the Pinot Grigio. As my blood sugar sinks lower, my body begins to lose control. I begin to feel so weak and lethargic that any basic movement, like shifting in my chair, feels like it takes ten times more energy than it normally does. I lose concentration, can't completely remember the last thing I said and can't properly follow the thread of conversations. This is the moment when I absolutely *have to* eat food that will lift the sugar level of my blood *very fast*. During this stage any food tastes extremely good. If I don't eat then I head rapidly into Stage 3.

Stage 3: Not funny. The not funny stage is absolutely as it sounds. This is when my blood sugar has sunk so low that I must *very urgently* be treated with some sugar-lifting food. This is where blood glucose goes so low that glucagon injections need to be used. By now, I will feel very lightheaded, dizzy, weak and tired. There is very little I can manage other than to sit and wait until the injection begins to work. This is the one and only time when diabetics might faint. So far, I am glad to say, it has never happened to me.

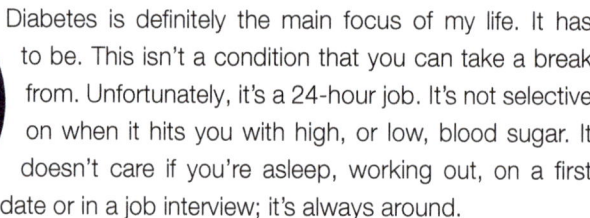

Diabetes is definitely the main focus of my life. It has to be. This isn't a condition that you can take a break from. Unfortunately, it's a 24-hour job. It's not selective on when it hits you with high, or low, blood sugar. It doesn't care if you're asleep, working out, on a first date or in a job interview; it's always around.

It's a big challenge, but there is a huge benefit in being able to accept that and get on with it. Don't get me wrong, there are times when it's very difficult, but as long as you treat it accordingly and don't neglect the severity of it, you can live a normal life.

Diabetes has changed a lot of that for me. Over the past few years it has consumed my life, but in a strangely good way. I've learned so much about the condition and a lot about myself. I've met and spoken to people who have been diabetic for twenty years, five years or just a few weeks.

I've changed my own perspective and my dream now is to change the world's perspective of diabetes.

Eoin Costelloe, personal trainer and model, Ireland

NIGHT-TIME HYPOS

Low blood sugar at night is a constant worry for Type 1s. After all, you won't be awake for the early 'fun' stage. These night-time lows take the average diabetic 100 per cent out of their routine. If you've not experienced one, allow me to describe what it is like. Imagine the following scene: you're fast asleep, dreaming and enjoying your night. Then, without warning, something that seems to be very similar to the feeling of your high blood glucose monster jolts you into consciousness. But this monster is sassier and loves ringing a bell. You quickly realise that the bell is not coming from the rest of the house, because that is enveloped in total silence, but rather from inside your head. You'll also notice that not only is it 2 or 3am, but the bell is showing no signs of respecting the crushingly early hour. Years ago, I might very well have been irritated by my noisy inner guest. However, I have grown to love this little banshee. It's telling me to wake up and make sure it is satisfied. As soon as I eat something, the sassy noise goes quiet. I will soon feel back to normal, certainly within ten to fifteen minutes, and, all being well, will return to my dream shortly thereafter. The only time I allow myself to become just a tiny bit irritated is when I can't get back to sleep. But really, it's fine. I've become used to it and am very grateful to my inner trespasser for letting me know about the upcoming emergency.

Things occasionally do get out of control, but there is little point having negative thoughts and cursing the fact you have Type 1. You can't change it. What you *can* change, however, is how you think about your situation, by sorting out your blood glucose levels pronto before they become serious. Train your brain to ignore negative emotions such as guilt, sadness, frustration or anger. By doing so, you will break the constant cycle of being stressed, anxious and depressed.

> I feel, overall, things have changed in a positive way for me since being diagnosed. I'm a big believer in the fact that you don't have any control over the things that happen to you in your life, but you do have control over how you react and respond to certain things. Type 1 is just bad luck. I never wanted to just lie down and feel sorry for myself – there are people a lot worse off than me.
>
> *Eoin Costelloe, personal trainer and model, Ireland*

Yes, you can!

I used to be a perfectionist when it comes to my blood glucose levels. I'd do impulsive insulin corrections and then… whop! See my blood glucose on the other edge of the range. This left me angry and feeling absolutely out of control. People around me could immediately tell that I was having an impulsive blood glucose day. Then, when browsing how others were coping, I read a very useful quote on Lauren Bongiorno's web page that said something like, 'The point is not to stay in range, but to stay in control.' I'd never viewed it in that way before. I was always focused on staying within the *perfect* numbers. I learned that, even if I am staying within range but have a roller-coaster-like blood glucose that needs constant involvement, then that is not *me* being in control. My blood glucose is. On the other hand, even if I am outside the borders, if the numbers are steady and predictable, I am the boss of the circumstances.

In the beginning, I was very shy with my diabetes. I never told people about it unless somebody needed to know, such as a school nurse, or classmates, or my teachers, but that was about it. Then, I realised that I couldn't do that any more because, when people didn't know I had diabetes, it made me constantly anxious. I knew that if something were to happen, nobody would know about it, or what to do, and my life could be at risk. After joining the online community, I became a lot more comfortable with sharing my disease publicly to whoever follows me. That's made me think more deeply about it and made it a lot more comfortable for me. Now, I'm fully comfortable sharing this part of my life as it is. Like it or not, it is probably the biggest part of my life. It's the one thing that determines my day and it's the one thing that affects what I can and cannot do at the moment.

In the last year, when I created a project (on diabetes) for my graphic design programme, that's when I fully accepted that I do have diabetes and that if people know about it, it's not the end of the world. My classmates slowly started to pick up that this disease is real and that this disease affects me in all of my work. But, with that, they also started asking me more questions about diabetes and how it affects me, how a different pump or a CGM (continuous glucose monitoring device) affects a person and what they do for different people. All of those moments helped me to realise that, yeah, I have diabetes, but this is like my *superpower*. It's something that defines me and makes me different from everybody else, but in a positive way. Yeah, I have a disease, but I can spread awareness and bring communities together. I felt like that is something that makes me unique in a good way.

David Mina, graphic designer, USA

BLOOD GLUCOSE DIARY

What does it really mean to have a predictable blood glucose? It is when it reacts to your actions as you'd expect. These expectations are drawn from your past experiences. Tracking your experiences, actions and reactions becomes much easier with a blood glucose diary. The diary typically involves noting your blood glucose levels at certain times of the day and stating how much you ate, how much insulin you injected and what activities you performed. It helps you to spot patterns and adjust next time you are faced with a similar situation.

I was forced to use a blood glucose diary early on. I won't lie, it was the last thing I wanted to do while trying to get on with my life and work towards my ambitious goals. Yet, whenever I saw control slipping out of my hands, I knew those notes I made would help me to discuss the patterns with my endocrinologist and, together, we always managed to agree on the next steps. After that, I was always better equipped to proceed with my endeavours with perfect blood glucose levels by my side.

You might hear something very similar *at least* another couple of hundred times from your healthcare team, who will stress just how important a blood glucose diary is. I too would like to emphasise that a blood glucose diary is a powerful tool for becoming more self-aware, recognising patterns and effectively treating yourself.

If you wonder where to get one, your medical team will probably have plenty in stock since they are regarded as a very common and effective tool in diabetes management. You might even find one online to print out for yourself.

Yes, you can!

CONTROLLING A HIDDEN DISEASE

Type 1 is essentially a hidden disease. The fact that you don't look ill can be a handicap sometimes. People will treat you as though you are entirely normal, even when you feel anything but. Occasionally, diabetes breaks out and doesn't react like you'd expect. Unfortunately, when we are out of control, it is easy for others to dismiss our symptoms as us being drunk. Whether we are telling terrible jokes or slumped in a chair looking disorientated, these are classic signs of having one too many. It is not an unusual sight when young people are out and about and there is nothing about our appearance that says, 'Actually, this person has Type 1 – please help.' This is why it is so important that at least one friend with you knows and understands your condition. However, your friend won't always be there. They may nip to the loo or get waylaid talking to someone else on the other side of the bar. In this case, paying attention to your body's signs is crucial. It means you don't have to be entirely reliant on the help of others. And this is where self-awareness comes in handy. It helps to know your body well enough to catch any unexpected blood glucose behaviour on time and take timely action (for example, eat before you get into a really bad hypo).

It is a true mental challenge to get used to the fact that your blood glucose levels do sometimes go outside the ideal range. Often we need to let things go and, instead of hating ourselves, accept it, analyse it, draw conclusions about further treatments and learn to work with the situation.

Keeping your diabetes under control mentally, physically and emotionally is something we all learn over time. Controlling your blood glucose levels will become part of your day-to-day schedule. Sometimes, staying in control can be as easy as, say, making a morning walk part of your daily routine. It's a great way to clear your mind, take some fresh air and just enjoy nature. Some of the wonderful participants in this book are experts in the fields of yoga and mindfulness, so if you are interested in controlling your blood glucose levels by using these techniques, I suggest you follow Drew, Evan or Lauren. Their daily social media content is filled up with professional advice in this field.

Mind, Body And Soul

I'd say to any Type 1 that what is really important is to stay positive and not to feel as though you are a victim, because that doesn't help anybody. I do realise that it's really easy to feel quite isolated. I didn't know any other Type 1s at university, or in my first few jobs, or anywhere around me at all. However, it's really useful to remember that there is actually a community out there. If anyone needs help, they can get it. They're not on their own. They also need to realise that, even when they have had a really bad day, it doesn't mean they've done something wrong. You know, everyone is allowed to have a bad day. Everyone is allowed to splurge on ice cream every now and then and it doesn't mean you're a bad person just because your bloods aren't good.

My ambition now, and this might sound really strange, is just to be content. I spent a lot of my youth chasing a career and wanting to be in the right area of work, with bigger and better jobs, with better pay and all these sorts of things. And then you reach a point where you start thinking about how to retire, which is scary because it happens so quickly. Now I am actively planning for retirement in maybe 15 or 20 years, my mindset is focused on wanting to have a happy and healthy life. I really just want to be content. It might sound a bit dull and boring, but I'm a great believer in having a sense of contentment. As Type 1s, we can take a very active role in staying well, rather than just leaving it to chance.

Stephen Dixon, Sky News presenter, UK

FEELING WORRIED? IT'S OK

Some days it's OK to let your diabetes go. You don't have to feel like a superhero every day. This makes you a completely normal person who has been diagnosed with diabetes and doesn't mean you have failed. It's also worth pointing out that some days, the best way to manage diabetes might be to watch a movie and eat your favourite food in bed. Life is too short to not listen to your body.

Sara Mobäck, influencer, Sweden

Yes, you can!

As Lauren noted at the opening of this chapter, it is not common practice for the healthcare system to pay holistic attention to issues related to diabetes. Therefore, in a chapter advocating the upsides of greater self-awareness, something I would like to touch upon is anxiety and depression. The experience of feeling low has largely remained an unaddressed topic in the treatment of diabetes. In the hospital where I was first diagnosed and treated, it was never discussed. As a result, no one really spoke about the mental impact and even my parents didn't consider that it might be mentally hard for me. I know that hospitals elsewhere often ignore the psychological wellbeing side when they advise on treatments too. In my case, the result was that my parents occasionally wondered why was I so 'emotionally unstable' at times when I had bad blood glucose levels. The whole family now know it is truly natural at certain times. You are perfectly normal if you experience some hardships. The good thing is, these low moments can be avoided.

Nearly everyone I spoke to for this book alluded to moments when their diagnosis had pulled the rug out from under them and they had felt really low. While these people have all gone on to find themselves and do what they want to do with their lives, with many becoming fantastic Type 1 ambassadors, any negative thoughts can't simply be ignored. Being told you have Type 1 comes as a real shock to anyone, and it is natural to feel worried about treatment, lifestyle changes and many more variables besides. It's a perfectly normal reaction and if that is how you are feeling now, you are not alone.

The advice here is designed to counter many of the negative emotions that you may feel. Understand, though, that you are not alone and can seek help from many different sources. One of the most important of these is the extremely powerful online community. However, I would urge everyone to be on their guard and watch out that their worries don't spill over into genuine anxiety and depression. By this, I mean over and above the day-to-day stresses of learning how to cope with a new and unfamiliar routine of counting carbs and measuring insulin levels. Symptoms of real underlying issues vary from person to person, but ones to watch out for include feelings of danger, panic or dread; rapid breathing; increased sweating; insomnia; obsessive behaviour; and difficulty focusing on anything other than what you are worried about. In some cases, anxiety can turn into panic attacks, which are sudden, intense episodes

Mind, Body And Soul

where people feel genuine fear despite there being no imminent threat or danger. Just to confuse matters, panic attack symptoms mimic those of a hypo. Attention and action are the best friends of a responsible diabetic. Speak to your diabetes team, as soon as possible, if you experience some or all of these symptoms.

In the beginning, I struggled a bit, feeling alone with this disease, and had a lot of depression. I had no zest for life and cried myself to sleep on many nights. I felt like I was the only one living with diabetes at the time because I didn't know anyone else who had this disease. I thought no one could understand. I developed a bit of a negative lifestyle and took up some bad habits. When I was about 13 or 14, my doctor told me I really need to take control of my health because, if I didn't, there would be some complications as a result. I realised that I had messed up a bit. I had to change my whole view of this disease.

I forced myself to look at everything. I put myself on a strict diet and exercise programme, and I joined the online diabetic community as well. This meant I was able to connect with people across the world who also live with diabetes. That has helped me in multiple ways. I always tell people that if it weren't for the online community, I really don't know where I would be at this point in my life. As soon as I met others living with diabetes, my depression completely went away. I felt like I was not the only one and I was not alone any more. It just changed my whole perspective on life, to the point where now I'm always saying how *good* life really is, despite this disease. I am so grateful that I can wake up every day and do what I get to do, every day, particularly with the online community. It's become my job at the moment and, as I often say, it is the best job I ever had. I'm able to connect with people and create fun and informative content for others to see. It helps them, but it also helps me. Sometimes I even forget that I have diabetes when I'm doing the work that I love.

There are definitely still moments when I feel like diabetes is going to get in the way of something that I want to do, or it is going to be challenging. But I always remind myself that diabetes can't own me and it can't win every time. I need to prove myself and others wrong when it comes to diabetes getting in the way. I tell myself, 'No, you want to do something, go do it. Diabetes can still be there, but you just will need to find a way to make it work.'

I love that feeling of accomplishing something, and then looking back and thinking, *remember when you told yourself you couldn't do something because of diabetes? Well, look at yourself now!* Diabetes is very tough and there are some dark moments, but it is the good moments that you need to focus on.

My advice to anyone is: reach out to other people with this disease, ask questions, and seek friendships, meet-ups and events. It will not only change your perspective on diabetes, but on life too.

David Mina, graphic designer, USA

Please remember: it is absolutely normal if things occasionally feel like they are getting out of control. The key to your happy life with diabetes is reacting on time to regain control. This might mean re-evaluating your actions on your own, or turning to your diabetes team for help. Even though diabetes is our own responsibility, we don't necessarily need to solve everything on our own. When you feel you can't cope, don't hesitate to ask for help. Diabetes management can easily become a fun team task once you find the team to discuss it with, whether that's your endocrinologist, family or friends, or a combination of all three.

10
ADVICE FOR PARENTS
OF CHILDREN WITH
TYPE 1 DIABETES

Yes, you can!

To say that I was shocked to find out that my child had diabetes would be an under-statement. When a child becomes diabetic, the life of a family changes in an instant. Parents are faced with questions about what to do, how to live and how to help their child.

Kristina was born completely healthy and literally did not get sick until she was 3 years old. She'd always been a very agile child and it was almost impossible to make her sit in one place. Then, suddenly in December 2000, just before Christmas, I began to notice that she had become sluggish and was sitting down more or lying on the couch. In the months before, she had grown a lot, so we hadn't really noticed that she had lost a lot of weight.

We went to see a paediatrician, who, after examining Kristina, told me everything was fine with her and maybe it was some kind of a virus. I calmed down a little, but not for long. Over the next week, her symptoms increased every day. She became even more sluggish, slept a lot, drank water constantly and got up to go to the toilet many times at night. She also began to eat a lot, which at first made me happy, because at one time it was a bit of a problem to feed her. Soon, though, I realised that, despite the abundant eating, Kristina was constantly hungry. Once again, we called our family doctor. He confirmed his earlier diagnosis – a viral infection. By now, I was convinced this was wrong. I have a medical background and had begun to suspect that this could be diabetes. But how could my child get diabetes? There was no history of diabetes in either my family or my husband's family. The next day, we went back to the hospital, taking some urine we'd collected in advance. The doctors in the emergency room looked at me in disbelief when I presented it to them, but they produced a test strip for checking the amount of sugar in the urine. My worst fears were realised. The tests showed the presence of acetone! Kristina was immediately hospitalised and put on a drip while all necessary tests were done. Her blood sugar at the time of admission was 52 mmol/L (over 900 mg/dL), compared a norm of up to 5.5 mmol/L (99 mg/dL). The attending physician

Advice For Parents Of Children With Type 1 Diabetes

announced the diagnosis – diabetes mellitus.

It took me a week to come to my senses and absorb the diagnosis. There was very little information on childhood diabetes available. These were the days before the internet, and I couldn't find any books about it. It was as if it did not exist at all. And we desperately needed support at that time – any information or the benefit of someone's experience!

At the time, no one uttered a word about healthy eating. I came to the conclusion that what is good for a diabetic is also good for healthy people, so the food intake and regime in our family changed, and we fully adapted to what Kristina ate. To this today, we still adhere to this diet.

In the search for alternative methods of treatment, we travelled to another city for acupuncture. Kristina's sugar was very low when this treatment was going on. However, I later realised that what I considered to be a miracle cure actually coincided with the so-called 'honeymoon period' of Type 1, a brief but small remission.

We had to change a lot of our plans. I had been intending to put Kristina in a kindergarten and go back to work. But now my days were spent constantly measuring sugar and insulin injections, calculating carbohydrates and preparing the right food. We also did brisk walks two times a day. When Kristina's metabolism returned to normal, she would be agile once more, but we constantly had to catch her blood sugar so that it did not fall too low. I got exhausted by what was going on in the daytime, but I had to measure her blood sugar while she was sleeping at night and feed her when hypoglycaemia occurred. Of course, the availability today of round-the-clock monitoring devices makes life much easier for children and their parents. Medicine is definitely advancing and that is encouraging.

Now Kristina is a grown woman and a student at Cass Business School in London, she lives an independent life and carefully controls her diabetes. She reads a lot and follows the latest updates on diabetology. My daughter knows very well that diabetes is not an obstacle to a fulfilling life and achieving her goals. On the contrary, Type 1 diabetics are accustomed to discipline from childhood. They quickly become self-sufficient and are able to control themselves like no other individuals.

The main task of parents in this situation is to teach diabetic children to live a full life. They should help them not to be embarrassed by their disease or to limit themselves to some kind of framework. They should teach them how to eat properly, systematically engage in sports, and control their diabetes with sugar measurements and insulin therapy. Do all of this and our children will live a long and happy life.

And one more important detail. Find the right doctor. We have been lucky, throughout the entire period of the disease, starting from when Kristina was 3 years old to this day, to be under the care of the same amazing endocrinologist, Dr Almássy Zsuzsanna. I thank her for her kindness, attention and professional competence.

Tatiana Loskarjova, Kristina's mum

It might seem like I've mentioned my parents a lot in this book, maybe even too much for someone who has reached their twenties. This is perhaps because they've played a huge role in my life when it comes to the topic of diabetes. They were the ones who helped me form my understanding of good treatment and shaped my attitude to the condition. (And, of course, I love them!) It is for this reason that I thought it helpful to end the book by writing about some of what I have learned that might be of help to parents who find themselves in a similar situation to mine.

My parents never sought to do anything to hold me back. Quite the opposite in fact. They encouraged me to live a very full and active life and, if I was ever inclined to put my feet up, they'd come up with a new activity to try. In the earliest years, they helped me manage my blood sugar levels and eat good food, and then, as I grew older, they encouraged me to be independent and make my own decisions. Mind you, as in any family, there were times when they weren't entirely sure of what I was up to, or they would surely have stepped in and offered a few words of wise advice. I am thinking in particular of the time when I embarked on a six-hour roller-skating trip into the centre of Budapest at the age of 11.

It was a hot summer's day and my childhood best friend, Diana, and I were spending a lot of time outside. In particular, we were doing a lot of roller skating, which was my favourite activity at the time. As 11-year-olds without smartphones (and consequently without Google Maps!), we always stuck to safe routes around our home to make sure we didn't get lost. One day, I had the brilliant idea of heading over to Heroes' Square, one of the most recognised tourist spots in Budapest, 10 km away from where we lived. That would be fun, right? The only slight issue was the fact that my parents had always been scared to let me travel alone on public transport or to go for long walks. They thought I was still a bit young. I decided not to tell them about my great idea.

'I have a sure plan,' I told Diana confidently. 'We always take the same route there by car. I know the way. It's easy, we'll be fine.'

I felt like a conqueror as we headed off at 8am. I had told my parents that I was going to a friend's house to play PlayStation. Everything seemed to be straightforward, literally. The car route was absolutely ramrod straight. Suddenly, though, we got to a point where pedestrians could not continue beside the road. *No worries*, we thought, *we'll find another route*. We took it as a challenge as we searched for the pedestrian routes running parallel to the road leading to the city centre. We weren't terribly successful, not least because we were in absolutely unknown territory, without a map, and it didn't help that the view of the familiar main road was frequently hidden among a maze of tall buildings.

My blood glucose was dropping low. Two hours into our trip, we had no idea how far we'd travelled or how much of our journey we had left. It was getting hotter and hotter too. Summers in Hungary can be really devastatingly hot and it was one of those true summer days.

Eventually, after four hours of travel time, we found our way to Heroes' Square. I felt like a true warrior. It was such a beautiful moment getting there without the accompaniment or help of an adult! I felt so independent. Of course, then I realised that we needed to complete the same route, backwards. It was midday, the sun was quite strong and my blood glucose was sinking lower. Still, though, I was super-happy and already on my third ice cream. Amazingly, we made the return trip in two hours and it was a moment of pure joy. I was so excited and proud for completing the six-hour trip! I couldn't help but tell the entire story to my parents and show them a picture of myself at Heroes' Square. The reaction was not at all what I expected. They were definitely not as excited as I was. Not even close. In my defence, I would say that this 'exercise' had a huge impact on my 11-year-old body. My blood glucose levels were absolutely perfect for quite a few days after the conquering of Heroes' Square! I should also add that, since that day, Diana has preferred to ignore me every time I have said, 'I have a sure plan.'

It is such a delicate moment when your child is diagnosed, even though we knew about diabetes because I had it myself. My wife and I were overwhelmed with the diagnosis itself and with all the information that we were given at once from the nurses, doctors and nutritionists. All the different insulin regimens. I really think the most important thing is to try to calm down and care for the parents, because when a child is diagnosed, they are the ones that will act like the 'pancreas'.

The most important task of a parent raising a child with diabetes is to help them face the condition in as natural a way as possible. I also tell my son that diabetes won't stop him pursuing any dream he has, just as it did not stop me. Diabetes is just a condition. It doesn't define us. Other people have other conditions and ours is diabetes.

Today we are diabetes buddies. He is proud of all his devices (continuous glucose monitoring device and pump) and tells everyone about them. Priceless.

Miguel Paludo, champion racing driver,
Brazil, and father to Oliver, also Type 1

CONFIDENCE AND CURIOSITY RULE

Even though Miguel has Type 1 himself, he found the moment his son Oliver was diagnosed difficult, just like my parents, who knew nothing about diabetes. However, while approaching it from different sides, they both came to the same conclusion. They realised that the best thing they could do for their child was to encourage confidence and curiosity about the world, while also making sure their child was safe. If you think about it, though, this goes for any parent really, whether of a Type 1 child or otherwise. In the early days, there might be a bit more work than usual, particularly if a family is entirely new to diabetes, but there is plenty of information out there now.

Advice For Parents Of Children With Type 1 Diabetes

My parents had their work cut out with me. I was an incredibly active young child. My brother and I were always larking around and doing sports together too. We'd play everything from classical games like badminton, table tennis and trampolining to more innovative ones like karate jumps. To my parents' credit, they never once tried to intervene. Nor should they have done on the grounds of my Type 1. But maybe they should have on the grounds of my brother's communication skills! He was especially keen on karate and one time, when the 17-year-old him was practising slow karate kicks, the job of the 7-year-old me was to move away from them. The next stage of the exercise was when he asked me to stay seated while he moved on to do his fast, full-speed kicks. Misunderstanding his instructions, I jumped right into his well-trained kick. His foot connected with my head, my head connected with the wall and I was knocked unconscious. I woke up in hospital surrounded by my very worried family. Fortunately, no long-term damage was done and I was allowed to go home the day after.

Another time, when I was 13, I decided to prove to my friends that I could skip with a skipping rope, non-stop, 500 times. I successfully completed the challenge. However, the result of my efforts was also a swollen ankle and instructions from the doctor to stay off my left leg for three months! This also meant I had to be home schooled. Home schooling was not a big problem for me, but the inability to walk was. My friends and I came up with loads of fun games that only involved my upper body (table tennis, various ball games and even knee-height boxing!). I didn't think about it much then (what kid does?) but, looking back, it was all more stuff for my parents to worry about. Again, though, they never once stepped in and said, 'Slow down, Kristina.' Perhaps they should have for my own safety. I have an impressive list of injuries. I spent two months with both arms in plaster after my love of headstands ended abruptly at the age of 10. I had a broken chin thanks to my love of running and a huge number of bruises. I lived it all!

Today, thinking back to moments like this, I keep on smiling. These are wonderful childhood memories that are part of the lives of most active kids. They really show that we, diabetics, are just normal kids with the ability to enjoy every part of life and live it to the full just like everyone else. I am very grateful to my parents for helping me to see that.

Yes, you can!

On many occasions throughout the years, Jonny would tell me that he had run out of strips for his tester, but it was worse when it was insulin he had run out of! It was a case of phoning the doctor, getting the prescription and picking it up from the chemist. Working as a child carer and with three kids in tow, it was sometimes very difficult and time consuming to organise this while he was at school, or at work, or rehearsing. I was always at the end of the phone to help, though. While it made me so mad at times, there was no way I would not sort it out for him. Being his mum, I wanted to make sure he stayed fit and well and that was my job. I do remember one time when he phoned me from a cabaret rehearsal saying he had no insulin. It was a Saturday evening, followed by Sunday and a bank holiday Monday and everything in Jersey (where we lived) was shut! I had to pull a lot of favours and phone calls to work out how to get the drugs, which I knew he needed urgently as he was rehearsing all day and using up a lot of energy in the routines. Mum to the rescue and the situation was thankfully sorted.

I cannot recall how many insulin pens he has lost either. That was his biggest fault. But he does look after himself and never forgets to take the insulin. He has always taken his condition very seriously.

I can understand why Jonny doesn't always tell me sometimes when he has a 'diabetic incident', as I would probably worry about him a lot more. Now he's fully grown and drinking regularly when socialising, it is expected, but you can't keep a mum from worrying. I am immensely proud of Jonny and how he copes with diabetes every day. He is a true role model to others. He even wrote a song about having the condition. He thought at one point that having diabetes might cost him his career in performing and TV. Now, I think *not*!

Collette Labey, Jonny Labey's mum

A lot of diabetes websites are information resources that focus on the shock of the diagnosis and the ways parents can help with insulin regimes and diet. This is all very important, especially if a child is very young

Advice For Parents Of Children With Type 1 Diabetes

when Type 1 becomes a part of their life. Parents also play an equally important part in helping their children achieve their full potential. Sometimes, as all the parents here note, this will entail a bit of gritted teeth as they watch their children take a few chances, but again, isn't that what good parenting is all about? Parents equip kids with all the tools they need to live a good life and let them get on with it with all their support. And a little bit of humour along the way too.

When I first got diagnosed and was prescribed my insulin, I was with my brothers and my mom. As we drove off afterwards, one of my brothers said, 'Let's go celebrate.' As it happened, there was an Olive Garden restaurant literally across the street.

As we were driving over, my brother asked, 'Do you think we should go and pick up the insulin you got prescribed during the consultation?' At the time, we didn't know anything about insulin, so I was like, 'No I think we'll be fine!' Little did I know (then) that insulin would keep me alive, and that I needed it to keep my blood sugar in control whenever I ate something, especially food full of carbohydrates like you get in Italian restaurants such as Olive Garden. We ate everything on the menu and I came home to a blood sugar of 22.2 mmol/L (400 mg/dL) (very high). I was like, 'What's going on – why is this happening?'

My mom said, 'Well, maybe it's because you had a whole bowl of pasta! Of course your blood sugar is high.' We were just so uninformed. But the beauty of this story is that my brother went out of his way to take me out and celebrate, instead of mourning and being sad that I had been diagnosed. The whole family looked at it in that way. Their attitude was, 'Oh, you have been diagnosed with something – now we know what it is and it's something we can treat and take care of, that's fine.'

Ali Abdulkareem, blogger and job coach, USA

AFTERWORD

My most passionate hope is that, after reading this book, you will agree that life is equally exciting for everyone, including anyone with Type 1 diabetes. Yes, diabetes will change a lot of things, but it doesn't have to be for the worse. In fact, quite the opposite. You can do everything you've ever done and bravely plan to do a lot more than you had ever previously imagined.

Dream big. Be brave. Achieve your goals and enjoy the opportunities that this wonderful life has to offer. And then write to me and tell me all about them.

ACKNOWLEDGEMENTS

I know we can! And I would like to thank everyone who helped me with sharing this knowledge in the form of this book.

My parents, for their limitless love, support and encouragement since my earliest days, for showing me that we can all achieve whatever we devote our minds to. Without them, this book would not have been possible.

Ali Abdulkareem, Csilla Németh, David Mina, Drew Harrisberg, Elin Sandström, Eoin Costelloe, Evan Soroka, Jonny Labey, Collette Labey, Josu Feijoo, Kevin Stewart, Kornelia Mango, Lauren Bongiorno, Matt Collins, Miguel Paludo, Rob Howe, Sara Mobäck and Stephen Dixon for believing in this project and for finding the time in their busy schedules to share their priceless experiences to help fellow Type 1s.

Dr Almássy Zsuzsanna, head doctor of the Metabolic Department at Pál Heim National Institute of Paediatrics in Budapest, Hungary, for her curiosity, open-mindedness and tireless hours of work while ensuring that all Type 1s under her care feel informed, safe and fulfilled. For teaching me the techniques of diabetes management. And for providing constructive, professional feedback throughout the process of writing this book.

The production team of Yes, you can!, especially Teena Lyons (editor), Hazel Bird (copyeditor) and Catherine Murray (designer), for their genuine support, expert advice and professional approach, while shaping my enthusiastic drafts into a coherent, practical, readable and presentable book.

To Farkas Diána Fruzsina and Szabó Katalin, the 'early adopters', for being the first to believe in and work on the concept of the book, and for their encouragement since the very beginning.

And, of course, to all my family and friends, with whom I lived through all the experiences mentioned in the preceding pages, for helping me live and love life with Type 1 diabetes.

CONTRIBUTOR BIOGRAPHIES

I have included, as is usual, biographies of all the people who kindly contributed to this book. To make things a little more interesting, I have asked each one to tell me about their own unique superpower in their own words! I have also included links to their Instagram accounts (where they have them) and suggest you follow them. This group is incredible as Type 1 opinion formers and their posts are part of the buzzing diabetes social media community.

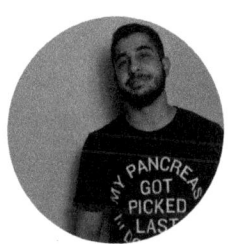

ALI ABDULKAREEM,
Blogger and job coach, USA –
@ali.abdlkareem

Ali is 23 years old and an Iraqi American living in San Diego, California. He migrated to San Diego in 1999 with his two older siblings from Baghdad, Iraq. Ali has been living with Type 1 diabetes for nearly six years following his diagnosis at the age of 18. He has a YouTube channel called The Diabetes Daily Hustle, which documents his everyday life with Type 1 diabetes, including working out, eating and just his everyday life with diabetes. He currently attends community college while pursuing other ventures.

Ali *can* because:
- Diabetes has taught me **self-awareness**. I believe diabetes doesn't change us, but rather exposes who we are. I realised my flaws, which showed up in the way I care for myself with regard to diabetes.
- Diabetes has taught me the **importance of health** and pushed me to learn beyond what the doctors told me to do. I have a large curiosity for fitness and the different foods that affect my mind and body. Diabetes gave me the purpose of developing an ongoing healthy relationship with food and exercising.
- Diabetes taught me **empathy** – empathy to understand that other people have their own journey and their own struggles. I must not

judge others because I must focus on my journey. My struggle from diabetes opened my eyes to other hardships around me.

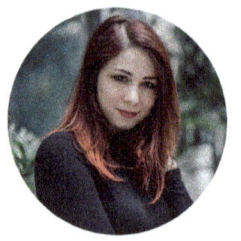

CSILLA NÉMETH,
influencer, blogger and photographer,
Hungary – @csillszvlog

Csilla is from Budapest, Hungary, and was diagnosed with diabetes at the age of 28. She is a beloved YouTube vlogger who actively documents her life and talks about fashion, make-up, food and portrait photography. You can see new videos at @csillszvlog on a weekly basis, with an audience spread far beyond the Type 1 community.

Csilla *can* because:

- I've come to love sports. Before diabetes I could never force myself to do any kind of physical activity!
- Now I know much better what I eat, and what foods are better for our bodies in general.
- I'm not scared of needles any more.

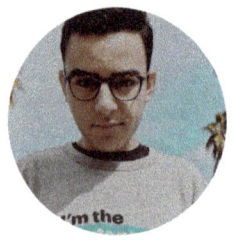

DAVID MINA,
Graphic designer, USA – @type1livabetic

David is from sunny California and was diagnosed with Type 1 diabetes back in 2008, at the age of 11. He is a creative graphic designer as well as a student going to school, studying to become a Certified Diabetes Educator. On Instagram, his main goal is to connect others in the community and promote a positive lifestyle as a young diabetic. In his free time, you will find David taking photos, riding his penny board or even taking a fun trip to Disneyland!

David *can* because:

Type 1 has shown me:
- How to be responsible.
- How to listen to my body.
- How to be more understanding.

Contributor Biographies

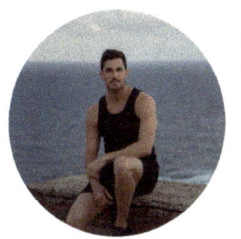

DREW HARRISBERG,
Physiologist, model and singer-songwriter, Australia – @drews.daily.dose

Drew is from Sydney, Australia, and was diagnosed with diabetes at the age of 22. Drew is an exercise physiologist, sport scientist, diabetes educator, model and singer – and, most importantly, he's a happy and healthy guy thriving with Type 1 diabetes. He is also a proud dog-father to his favourite dog, Dennis. Drew's main purpose is to teach others how to take control of their health so that, like him, we can live our best life! Drew developed a holistic 'Five Pillar' approach to empower individuals and guide them to a happy life. You can learn more about it on his website: drewsdailydose.com.

Drew *can* because:

Type 1 has shown me:
- How to turn adversity into opportunity.
- Passion, purpose and direction.
- Exercise is medicine.

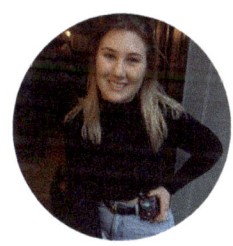

ELIN SANDSTRÖM,
Health and PE student and influencer, Sweden – @mylifewithdiabetes

Elin was born in 1996 and raised in Småland, in the south part of Sweden. She got her Type 1 diabetes in the year 2000, when she was 4 years old, and cannot remember a life without the disease. Elin has always had a positive attitude to her life with diabetes but recognises that this is a thing that not everyone has. Because of this, Elin likes to work with individuals who have diabetes and she is vice president of a federation for young people with diabetes, Young Diabetes Sweden, which provides youth diabetes camps and lectures about diabetes. Elin wants to spread a positive attitude! Besides that, she is studying health and physical education. In her spare time, she loves training, travelling and playing music.

Elin *can* because:

- I've learned to know my body from the inside and out.

Yes, you can!

- I've gained knowledge about health, nutrition, physical activity and the body.
- I've learned to take responsibility and never give up! I have diabetes, but diabetes doesn't have me.

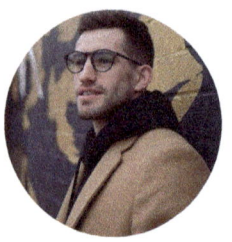

EOIN COSTELLOE,
Personal trainer and model, Ireland – @insuleoin

Eoin is a Type 1 diabetic from Dublin, Ireland. He was diagnosed at the age of 19 and, since then, diabetes hasn't just become part of his physical health; it's also shaped his life into what it is today and become his full-time job, which he couldn't be more happy about! He was named the Diabetes Male Fitness Influencer of the Year at the inaugural Diabetes Awards in Hollywood, California. He is an online diabetic personal trainer and fitness coach, working with diabetics all over the world to help them reach their full potential and ensuring that the condition does not control their mental or physical health. Eoin has also set up a diabetic podcast called *The insuleoin Podcast: Redefining Diabetes*. Every Wednesday he releases a new episode sharing his personal experiences with the condition and interviews.

Eoin *can* because:
- I've learned to value my health and never to take my health for granted.
- I live more consciously and enjoy every small moment – no matter how inadequate it may seem.
- I have to appreciate the amazing people and friends who have been brought into my life as a result of being diagnosed with diabetes, including those I never would have met otherwise.

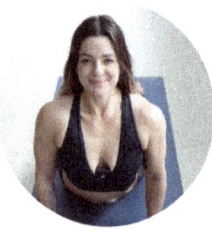

EVAN SOROKA,
Yoga therapist, USA – @evan_soroka

Evan was diagnosed with Type 1 diabetes in early adolescence and quickly found yoga as a tool to resolve the physical and mental challenges of diabetes. These experiences influenced her path as a therapist and healer. She has the highest qualifications in her field with a degree from the prestigious American Viniyoga Institute. Evan provides her clients with the skills to overcome health challenges, increase their self-awareness, and shift their attitude about their life and circumstances. Evan is the author of *Rise above Diabetes: A Yoga Therapy Manual*, coming out in 2021. She is also the owner of Soroka Yoga Therapy and a contributor to *Yoga International* and *Yoga Journal*.

Evan *can* because:
Type 1 has shown me:
- Compassion.
- Patience.
- Investigation.

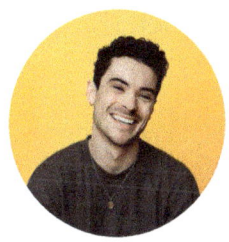

JONNY LABEY,
Actor, UK – @jonnylabey

Jonny is from the UK and was diagnosed with Type 1 at the age of 15. He is an English actor, dancer and singer. Jonny is known for playing a role in the famous British soap opera *EastEnders*, for being the original lead in a West End show called *Strictly Ballroom*, for participating in various TV shows (such as *The X Factor: Celebrity*) and for winning the *Dance Dance Dance* talent show. Jonny has recently started his own production company, NineByFive. In his free time, Jonny loves travelling, organising events and running his own diabetes blog, called *Know Your Type*.

Jonny *can* because:
Type 1 has helped me with:
- Good nutrition.
- Positive outlook.
- Determination.

169

Yes, you can!

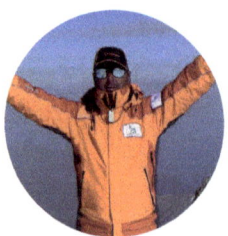

JOSU FEIJOO,
Mountaineer and astronaut, Basque Country - www.josufeijoo.com
Josu is a perfectionist – very meticulous, faithful and honest with his friends. He is ambitious and committed to achieving challenges. He does not like excuses. In fact, he says diabetes is not an excuse, it is just a travelling companion.

He says that the challenges he has faced – Everest, the great peaks, and his training in the various space centres where he has earned the titles of astronaut and cosmonaut – do not understand who is a diabetic and who is not. His philosophy is that you have to be responsible and only then will you get what you want. However, the 'lucky' factors must also be taken into account!

Josu can because:
Type 1 has helped me be:
- Very meticulous.
- Very strict.
- Responsible.

KEVIN STEWART,
publishing contracts consultant, UK
Kevin has lived in Kent for nearly 50 years. He was diagnosed with Type 1 at the age of 30, being told he had late onset juvenile diabetes. Kevin works in the field of publishing contracts, initially spending 20 years at one of the major UK publishers and subsequently setting up a consultancy, Contracts People, to support those needing expert advice. He has also been published in English (and, he has been told, Japanese) on the subject. Any spare time outside is spent walking, preferably to an obscure prehistoric site. Spare time inside is spent cooking and listening to increasingly obscure music.

Kevin can because:
Type 1 has helped me see:
- Diabetes is not a bad condition to have. There are so many worse things to suffer from. You can control diabetes.

Contributor Biographies

- By keeping records of what happens, you can probably do anything – you just need to plan first and learn from any consequences.
- The world is an absurd place that you cannot bend to your will. Life is pure chance. Enjoy it and seize the moments available.

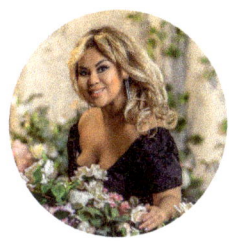

KORNELIA MANGO,
Singer and celebrity, Russia –
@korneliamango

Kornelia is a popular Russian singer, originally from Astrakhan, now living in Moscow. She is proud of her mixed blood – her dad is African and her mum is Tatar. Kornelia was diagnosed with diabetes at the age of 27. She is a professional singer and artist, has been a participant on famous Russian TV shows such as *The Last Hero* and *Cruel Games*, was a finalist in *The Star Factory* and won *Dancing with the Stars*. Today, Kornelia gives painting lessons, participates in music festivals and appears on various TV shows. Kornelia is the only famous diabetic in Russia who speaks openly about her diabetes. She encourages others with her lively lifestyle while actively blogging on YouTube and Instagram.

Kornelia *can* because:
Type 1 has helped me to:
- Be active.
- Make sure I love life because you never know what will happen next.
- Eat well.

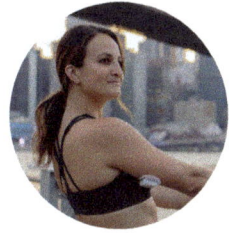

LAUREN BONGIORNO,
Diabetes health coach, USA –
@lauren_bongiorno

Lauren is a virtual diabetes health coach and creator of *The Diabetic Health Journal*. Living with Type 1 diabetes since 2000, she has coached hundreds of clients in her programmes and courses through her signature A1C Shift Method since 2015. Speaking across the USA as the Resident Diabetes Coach for Omnipod, she's been able to see what's missing in the traditional diabetes management model and fill that gap. Lauren's programmes and resources are rooted in her 360-degree approach, emphasising wellness throughout the mind and body. Lauren's success with client transformations and recognition as a coach in the community come from being an expert in initiating mindset and behaviour change, and also in providing the support and accountability outside the endocrinologist's office. Lauren was recently nominated by Pure Wow as one of the top 100 entrepreneurs to watch, for her impact in the diabetes space. You can visit her website at www.laurenbongiorno.com and connect with her on Instagram.

Lauren *can* because:
Type 1 has helped me see:
- The importance of self-awareness.
- The importance of self-sufficiency.
- The importance of self-compassion.

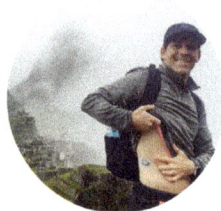

MATT COLLINS,
Robotic surgery business leader, USA – @matt_t1d

Matt was born in Mexico City, Mexico, and brought up in Bloomfield Hills, Michigan. He was diagnosed with Type 1 diabetes at the age of 15. He is now a medical device professional, father, husband and author of *T1D Pro*. Matt is currently in the process of relocating to Santiago, Chile, for work. He is expecting to be in South America for 18 months before returning to the States. In his spare time, Matt enjoys teaching his daughter new things, sports of all kind, and fly-fishing… he is yet to catch 'the big one'.

Matt *can* because:
Type 1 has helped me with:
- The understanding of food: to be honest, I'm not sure I would know anything about food if I didn't have Type 1. After diagnosis, however, I learned quite a bit – everything from how to read labels to types of foods and their effect on blood sugars and general performance.
- The importance of sleep: you never really know what 'tired' means until you've experienced the Type 1 roller coaster.
- Friendship! I've met a ton of really cool people around the world with Type 1 and I'm happy to call them my friends. It's been quite fun to go through everything we experience together!

Contributor Biographies

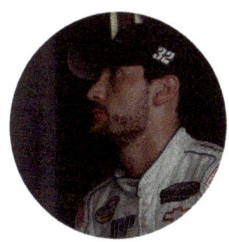

MIGUEL PALUDO,
Champion racing driver, Brazil –
@miguelpaludo

Miguel was born in Brazil and was diagnosed with Type 1 diabetes at 21 years old. He is a professional racing car driver and five-time champion in the Porsche Carrera Cup Brazil. Since his diagnosis, Miguel has enjoyed spreading awareness of diabetes through his social platforms. Miguel is married to Patricia Paludo and is the father of 8-year old Oliver Paludo, who has also been diagnosed with Type 1 diabetes, in his case at 8 months old. The family live in Mooresville, North Carolina.

Miguel *can* because:
Type 1 has helped me with:
- Patience.
- Healthier life.
- Self-knowledge.

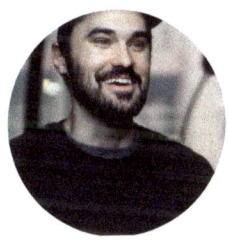

ROB HOWE,
Entrepreneur and founder, USA –
@robhowe21

Rob has been living with Type 1 diabetes for 15 years. He is an entrepreneur, marketing strategist, podcaster and former professional basketball player. In 2015, Rob founded Diabetics Doing Things in an effort to raise awareness around the amazing things that Type 1 diabetics are doing around the world. As of 2020, Rob's podcast has been downloaded over 1.5 million times by listeners in over 70 countries. Rob lives in Dallas, Texas, with his wife Erica and their fur babies, Michael J. Fox, Rowan and Enzo.

Rob *can* because:
- Diabetes has made me better at failure. When I don't get something right, I'm able to bounce back, just like people with diabetes do with their blood sugars.
- Diabetes has made me more present with my health, and understand the power of community.

Yes, you can!

- The diabetes community has introduced me to so many of my closest friends, colleagues and collaborators, and I'm truly grateful for that.

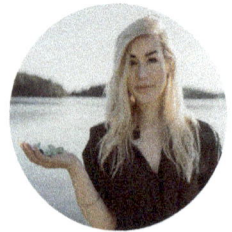

SARA MOBÄCK,
Influencer, Sweden – @saramoback

Sara writes one of Sweden's biggest blogs about Type 1 diabetes. She advocates a positive life despite a chronic illness, and realising your dreams, both big and small. This is something that is very important subject to Sara since she feels that many diabetics don't see the possibilities. In particular, she campaigns against the different types of guidelines for what we should eat and not eat. Because of this, and because the focus is more on our blood sugar curve and A1C levels (a test that shows average blood sugar level over the past two to three months), it can be difficult to know if a diabetic person has developed an eating disorder. Girls and women with Type 1 diabetes are twice as likely to develop an eating disorder as those without diabetes. Sara herself was diagnosed with anorexia nervosa in February 2017 and says it was one of the toughest periods in her life. She says her life goes up and down like everyone else's but today she is very positive and that helps her a lot.

Sara *can* because:

- Diabetes has taught me to be myself – being able to put myself first and think about what's best for me is a valuable strength.
- I am flexible and able to adapt to different situations when it comes with dealing with diabetes.
- Diabetes has taught me to take the positives from everything and any situations that can come together with diabetes. Being adaptable to new situations and circumstances is incredibly valuable because you never know what is around the corner in a long endurance race.
- Diabetes has taught me to remind myself that it is OK when things don't go to plan.

Contributor Biographies

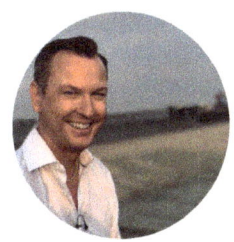

STEPHEN DIXON,
Sky News **presenter, UK –**
@stephendixontv

Stephen is a journalist and news presenter from the UK. He was diagnosed at the age of 17, just before heading to university. Stephen has always accepted Type 1 as part of who he is and firmly believes in embracing diabetes to get the best results.

Stephen *can* because:

Type 1 has helped me become:
- Conscious of all my health needs.
- Aware of what I eat (*this does not stop me having the odd tub of ice cream…!!*).

USEFUL SOURCES OF FURTHER INFORMATION:
Local Diabetes Organisations And Charities

Many of the websites of the leading diabetic organisations are mines of useful information. Several also have areas for member discussions, which are really helpful when it comes to sharing thoughts on certain issues or if you need further information. Four such sites that are definitely worth looking at are:

Beyond Type 1: https://beyondtype1.org
Diabetes.co.uk: https://www.diabetes.co.uk
International Diabetes Federation: https://idf.org
JDRF Type One Nation: https://forum.jdrf.org

AUTHOR BIOGRAPHY

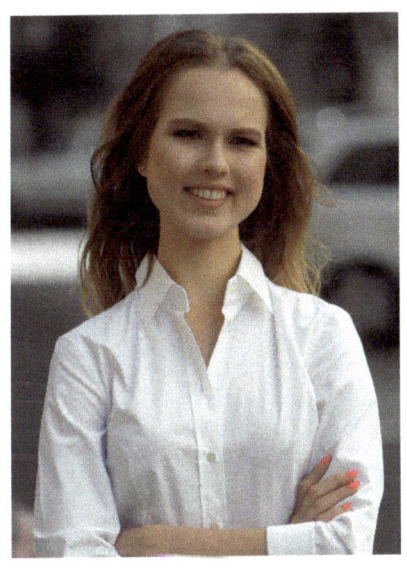

Kristina is a spirited businesswoman and author who was diagnosed with Type 1 diabetes at the age of 3. She considers herself lucky for having been raised by parents who believed she could do anything in life, regardless of diabetes. Kristina has enjoyed numerous exciting and buzzing experiences while successfully managing her diabetes and is now showing other Type 1s that this lifestyle, and indeed any chosen lifestyle, is possible. After moving to London at the age of 18, she began collecting success stories from individuals across the world with Type 1 diabetes. Her goal was to prove to others that anyone, anywhere with Type 1 diabetes can pursue their dreams. This book is the result of those inspiring conversations. Today, Kristina is still happily living in London, continuing to explore opportunities that this interestinglife has to offer while actively working on her business ventures.

You can follow her newest adventures and share your stories with her on Instagram (@kristinaloskarjova) or via email kristina@loskarjova.com

Yes, you can!

www.ingramcontent.com/pod-product-compliance
Lightning Source LLC
LaVergne TN
LVHW050059080526
838200LV00096B/390/J